ELLE & COACH

ELLE & COACH

Diabetes, the Fight for My Daughter's Life,
and the Dog Who Changed Everything

STEFANY SHAHEEN
with
MARK DAGOSTINO

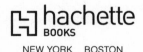

hachette
BOOKS

NEW YORK   BOSTON

Hachette Books
Hachette Book Group
1290 Avenue of the Americas
New York, NY 10104

www.HachetteBookGroup.com

Printed in the United States of America

RRD-C

First Edition: August 2015
10 9 8 7 6 5 4 3

Hachette Books is a division of Hachette Book Group, Inc.
The Hachette Books name and logo are trademarks of Hachette Book Group, Inc.

The Hachette Speakers Bureau provides a wide range of authors for speaking events. To find out more, go to www.hachettespeakersbureau.com or call
(866) 376-6591.

The publisher is not responsible for websites (or their content) that are not
owned by the publisher.

Library of Congress Cataloging-in-Publication Data

Shaheen, Stefany.
    Elle & Coach : diabetes, the fight for my daughter's life, and the dog who
changed everything / Stefany Shaheen with Mark Dagostino.
        pages cm
    ISBN 978-0-316-25876-0 (hardback)—ISBN 978-1-4789-0465-6 (audio
download) — ISBN 978-0-316-25874-6 (ebook) 1. Shaheen, Elle. 2. Diabetes
in children—United States. 3. Service dogs—United States. 4. Detector
dogs—United States. 5. Dogs—Therapeutic use—United States. 6. Human-
animal relationships—United States. 7. Shaheen, Stefany—Family. 8. Mothers
and daughters—United States. I. Dagostino, Mark. II. Title. III. Title:
Elle and Coach.
    RJ420.D5S53 2015
    615.8'5158083—dc23
                                                              2015019799

For the scientists who will one day find a cure and for all those who are working to make life better until then...

CONTENTS

First Glimpse

"Dogs are helpful to *some* people."
—"What Dogs Do for People"
by Elle, age 7

My phone buzzed on the kitchen counter and I hurried to pick it up. It was Craig, texting from Kansas.

"Here he is," Craig wrote. "And you'll never believe what his name is. His name is Coach!"

Coach? I thought. Of all the names in the world, the dog's name is Coach?

I opened the picture and laid eyes on that dog for the very first time: an adorable, floppy-eared yellow Lab, wrapped in the arms of my oldest child, Elle.

Elle? I thought. Dogs made Elle nervous. She'd been bitten twice in her short life. Yet there she was, happily hugging a dog that she'd only just met, a dog with deep brown eyes and the most expressive face.

My daughter not only looked happy, but she also looked *at ease*.

For months I'd questioned this decision. Were we really so desperate that my husband and daughter had to fly all the way to Kansas? Did we really believe that an animal could do things that neither Elle's doctors nor I had been able to do for her over the last five and a half years? Not to mention that I could hardly fathom how a dog might fit into our family's already-frenetic life.

Still, I couldn't stop smiling. My daughter was beaming—and I swear that dog was, too.

I really do hope this works, I thought. *For her sake. For my sake. For all of us.*

ELLE &
COACH

CHAPTER 1

The Diagnosis

"I was so scared. I actually thought that I was going to die."

—Elle, age 12

It was the Friday after Thanksgiving. We had already stuffed ourselves in the company of our extended family that Thursday, and we were counting our blessings as we set off on what we hoped might turn into a new tradition. My husband, Craig, and our four young children all piled into the minivan for two nights at the Mount Washington Resort, a historic grand hotel in New Hampshire's White Mountains, nestled at the foot of the Northeast's highest peak, with sweeping views of the entire Presidential Range. There was a chance for some fresh snow along with the warmth of an indoor pool, a promised visit from Santa Claus, and a plan to go pick out our Christmas tree that Sunday before we headed home. With Craig and I both working full-time, it was the first vacation we'd taken in ages, so the anticipation was palpable and the excitement radiated from all but one of us: my oldest daughter, Elle (which we pronounce "Ellie"). She did not share our enthusiasm, and I could not understand why.

Out of all the kids, Elle had always been the people pleaser. She had turned eight two months earlier, and I could hardly recall a time in her life prior to that September when she wasn't full of positive energy.

Elle was born with bright blue eyes and the biggest dimples anyone in our family had ever seen on a baby. It's as if she'd been smiling before she greeted the world. By the age of two, she started singing for anyone who cared to listen, dancing on tabletops or in the living room after insisting that we move the coffee table. A classic extrovert, she lived for applause, acceptance, and affection, whether it came from an audience of her parents, her teachers, her siblings, or perfect strangers. As she got older, she would often help clear the table or clean up her room without complaint, the first time we asked. She was loving and sensitive and cooperative. Our Elle. She wanted to make the people around her and the people she loved happy. Yet that night, on the way back to our room after a wonderful dinner complete with ice cream and capped off by a movie, Elle insisted that we all go swimming.

"We can't tonight," Craig said. "The pool's closed, but we'll go in the morning."

"No!" Elle shouted. "I want to go swimming *now*!"

She was belligerent. There was no reasoning with her. Our younger children accepted the reality almost immediately. After all, there was nothing we could do about the fact that the pool was closed. But Elle wouldn't let it go. The insolence wasn't like her.

For months she had seemed a little off to me, but I could not put my finger on what was wrong. She just wasn't herself. Ever since the start of the school year, she would cry at the drop of a hat, and when we asked her what was going on, she would say, "I just don't know what is wrong with me." I tried to convince myself it was a phase. She was getting older. Girls go through things. But it wasn't just tears and occasional mood swings. She started to struggle so badly in her math class that we received calls from her teacher. She wouldn't focus, her teacher said. She was fidgety. She frequently left to go to the bathroom. She kept complaining that she couldn't see the board, even after we moved her to the front row, and even after a routine eye exam confirmed that her vision was fine. She did poorly on her tests, too.

We'd never been called by one of her teachers with a concern, ever, until that fall. I just wasn't sure what was going on with my little girl.

Craig, my athletic husband with prematurely gray

hair, who had long ago earned the nickname "Silver Fox," wondered if she needed more time outside. He's someone who truly believes that fresh air, exercise, and time in nature can cure almost anything, so he used that gorgeous New Hampshire fall as a perfect excuse to get all four of our kids out in the sunshine as often as possible. Annah, our green-eyed athlete; Caraline, our brown-eyed budding comedienne; and William, the baby of the family, who had dimples just like Elle's, kept their summery, sun-kissed skin and rosy cheeks all season. So did Elle. It didn't seem to make a difference, though. She'd be fine one moment, then sobbing or snapping at her siblings the next.

All of it was troubling to me, but her attitude at the hotel that night was over the top. She was one notch shy of a full-blown tantrum over something that couldn't be changed. It made no sense.

Elle went to bed angry and complaining of a headache, and I lay down concerned.

Squeezing six people into one hotel room doesn't make for the best night's sleep, so I couldn't help but notice when Elle got up to go to the bathroom three times that night. That seemed strange to me, too.

We woke up first thing Saturday morning and took the whole gang to the pool before breakfast. Elle wore shorts and a T-shirt over her suit for the walk through the lobby, so I didn't notice anything unusual until we were poolside. Then, as she and the others were playing some game, I saw that her one-piece bathing suit was loose and puckering at the shoulders. It was nearly falling off her, and I knew it had fit just fine that summer. I had expected she would soon need a new suit that was the next size up, not *down*.

Why on earth would Elle be losing weight? I wondered.

She looked frail. The more I looked at her, the more her color seemed off, too. Elle looked almost gray. She had shadows under her eyes.

"Elle, are you feeling okay?" I asked her.

"Yes," she said, jumping back into the pool. She seemed annoyed that I'd asked the question. In fact, she seemed annoyed at everything any of us said or did the whole rest of that day. She kept barking at her siblings, even at William—her two-year-old brother whom all three of our girls mostly adored. Something wasn't right. She was sick. I was sure of it. As all of this went round and round in my mind, my instincts began pointing me toward something that seemed too far-fetched to believe.

Craig's younger brother, the kids' tall red-haired uncle Trent, had been diagnosed with type 1 diabetes in his twenties. I'd talked to him about the daily struggle of it all—the finger pricking, the insulin shots. I could hardly imagine how he put up with the demands of it. When I had asked him about the signs and symptoms that led to his diagnosis, he said he ate ravenously but kept losing weight; he ran to the bathroom all the time; he had headaches; he was tired; his thirst was unquenchable. Elle didn't have all of those things— at least, not all at the same time. She didn't complain of physical ailments or fatigue in a way that I would associate with something as serious as diabetes. She was thirsty a lot, but aren't all kids? I didn't think she was going to the bathroom multiple times per night on *most* nights. Just *last* night.

I tried to convince myself that I was being paranoid. But I couldn't shake it.

That night, Craig stayed in the room with the kids while I went down to use the computer in the hotel lobby. I started searching her symptoms on Google and WebMD. Sure enough, just about every symptom Elle exhibited—including irritability—pointed toward diabetes.

I barely slept that night. Elle woke up to go to the bathroom, twice. Both times she stopped to take a drink of water. A long drink. My stomach turned.

I whispered my suspicions to Craig, and he thought for sure I was overreacting. "Couldn't it be a virus?" he asked. "Maybe a urinary tract infection?"

Maybe.

So the next morning we started quizzing her.

"Does it hurt when you go to the bathroom?"

"No."

"Well, how long have you been this thirsty?"

"I don't know..."

She seemed annoyed, so we stopped. We gathered the kids, packed up the car, and headed over to the Rocks Estate, a stunning, 1,400-acre Christmas-tree farm full of rolling hills and old stone walls in the little town of Bethlehem.

Both Craig and I grew up in New Hampshire. Our roots here run deep. We still live within twenty minutes of most of our family members, just two hours south of that tree farm, in a small, historic city in the state's Seacoast Region, where the smell of the sea often permeates the air. In the North Country, where we'd both spent time as kids and were now returning with our own, the air was crisper and cleaner than just about anywhere else on earth. Craig made sure we all stopped and took a moment to breathe it in. That air made the hairs in my nostrils freeze, and the winters here often wore on me, but I had to admit, it was stunning. Fields of Christmas trees covered in a dusting of snow stretched as far as the eye could see. A horse-drawn cart pulled visitors down snowy paths, and the only scent besides fresh-cut pine was the smoke from a fire pit out behind the gift shop, where children gathered to roast marshmallows and make s'mores.

Craig and I were busy taking turns holding William and trying to keep track of our four- and six-year-olds,

Caraline and Annah, as they ran between the trees, laughing and fighting over which tree we should pick, when Elle told us she had to go to the bathroom.

"Hold on a minute," I said. "I'll walk back up with you."

That's when Elle had an accident. At eight years old, she wet her pants. She stood there in the freezing cold with her pants soaking wet, mortified. The look on Craig's face said it all: *What is going on?*

There were other people around who saw what happened. Elle saw them looking and started to cry. I hurried her to a bathroom near the gift shop to get her cleaned up and did my best to calm her down. Inside, I quietly panicked.

Cutting the day short, we picked out a tree as quickly as we could and immediately headed for home. During the two-hour drive, Elle grew nauseous. She complained of a headache again. I called our pediatrician's office and they told us to bring her in first thing the next morning.

I never went to bed that night. I stayed up checking on her, waiting anxiously for the sunrise.

～∞～

Our pediatrician's office was a few miles over the border in Maine. I called my brother-in-law Trent while I drove, praying that he'd tell me I was overreacting.

He didn't.

"It really sounds like type 1," Trent said, adding quickly, "but it could be something else. Let's just hold out hope."

From what I recalled, Trent's form of diabetes had no cure. I knew it could lead to serious complications if left untreated. I knew it required daily monitoring and care. It scared me.

Elle was no better, even after a good night's sleep. "Mom," she said as we pulled out of the driveway, "something's really wrong with me." She barely spoke the rest of the drive. She slumped down in her seat. She was weak. I almost had to carry her from the car into the office.

Dr. Westinghouse, a woman who had young kids of her own and who knew me and my children extremely well, is the type of doctor you won't find much anymore, one who would happily take my calls even on weekends when she was off duty. I trusted her. Unfortunately, she was out that day, so we saw someone else instead. I listed off Elle's symptoms and the timeline of the progression over the weekend and he gave her the once-over. "I'm worried that she might have diabetes," I said.

I told him about Trent's diagnosis and mentioned that I knew it could be hereditary.

"I don't think that's what this is," he responded. "It could be as simple as constipation."

Constipation? Seriously? I'd read that all it would

take to determine if Elle was diabetic was a urine test. So I asked him if she should be tested.

"I don't think that's necessary," he said.

"Can't we just rule it out?" I asked. *The test is simple*, I thought. From what I understood, it would take only a few minutes. It was an in-office test. If it showed sugar in her urine, then she had diabetes. If it didn't, then she might need further testing. But at least we'd know *something*.

"I'm *sure* that's not what this is," he said.

"Well, I hope you're right, but it's a simple urinalysis you can do right here in the office. Can you just do it? Please?"

"Well...," he said, "I'll do the urinalysis, but only to make you feel better."

"Thank you," I said. "Hopefully the test will confirm that I am wrong and I *will* feel better."

I took Elle to the bathroom. We handed over her sample.

Three minutes later, he returned to the examination room with his head down.

"It's positive," he said, staring at the floor. "She definitely has sugar in her urine. I'm going to get Dr. Westinghouse on the phone right away."

"How bad is it?" I asked.

"I don't know how elevated her blood sugar is right now," he said. "But it's conclusive. She's spilling sugar into her urine, which is a positive diagnosis."

"What?" Elle said. "What's wrong with me?"

"Elle," I said as calmly as I could. "I think you have diabetes. Like your uncle Trent has had for a few years. That's why you're feeling so sick."

She immediately saw through my attempt to stay calm and started to whimper.

"Mom, I'm scared," she said. She slid off the examination table and climbed into my lap. I put my arms around her, and despite how big she seemed compared to our little ones, in that moment she felt tiny. Fragile.

"It's going to be okay," I said. I didn't know whether I believed those words as I spoke them. I had so many questions: How long has she had this? Why did she get it? How can I possibly explain it to her when I don't understand it myself?

Dr. Westinghouse called in to the office a few minutes later. "I'm sorry about this news," she said. "It's going to be tough. It's going to be really tough. But it will get easier in time. Just know that, okay?"

"Okay," I said. Honestly, I had no idea what she was talking about. All I wanted were some instructions on how to make Elle feel better.

"I can either send you to Maine Medical or to Boston Children's," she said. She paused. "I know you, Stefany, and if I were in your shoes, I'd be in the car and on my way to Boston Children's right now. You'll have to be admitted through the ER, but I'll call ahead. Oh, and before you go, I need you to do lab work at

York Hospital. We need to know how high her blood sugar is before we can let you transport her safely."

I was surprised they couldn't test her right there in the office, but I agreed, and off we went. I called Craig. He was dumbfounded.

"She can't have it," he said. "She just can't." He was shocked. He couldn't believe it. I called Trent back, too. "No!" he said. He sounded dreadfully sad. His voice felt ominous to me. They both insisted on meeting us at York Hospital, which was just up the road.

"What's happening, Mom?" Elle asked as I tried to hurry her inside. "What do I have to do?"

"They need to run some tests. They're going to draw some blood for this one, okay? But you're tough. You can do this," I said.

Elle felt so miserable I think she would have gone along with almost anything at that point. But she didn't say much of anything at all. Her quietness worried me. *How bad is this?* I wondered.

Trent and Craig arrived at the hospital as we waited for her lab results. Their arrival calmed me a bit, until I looked at Trent. The sight of his face nearly buckled me. This six-foot-three man who looked so much like my husband could not hold back his tears. I didn't understand why he was so upset. He seemed to be living with diabetes just fine.

When the doctor came back with the results of Elle's blood work, the situation went from bad to worse. "She's very high," the doctor said. "You can't go home. You can't give her anything to eat. You need to go straight to Children's Hospital. Understand?"

So off we rushed down I-95 for the longest hour-and-a-half drive of our lives. No belongings. No instructions. No understanding of what would come next. Trent couldn't come with us. We didn't know how long we'd be staying. I called my cousin to ask if she could watch our three younger kids for the night if necessary, and she agreed.

The emergency room at Boston Children's Hospital was flooded with people. Everywhere we looked we saw sick kids. Dr. Westinghouse had done as she promised and called ahead. They got us into a room in the ER quickly so they could evaluate Elle immediately. A doctor ordered more lab work, and out came the needles. Elle took it like a trouper. *She's such a tough kid,* I thought. They started an IV, and she began to feel a little better, but the fluids forced her to go to the bathroom every fifteen minutes. She was shy about walking in her hospital gown. She wanted me at her side each time she went. So there we were, mother and daughter, pushing her IV pole to the public bathroom.

Finally the doctor came back into that tiny room with Elle's test results in hand. "You're not going to believe this," he said. "Her blood sugar is 964."

I had no idea what that number meant. "What *should* it be?" I asked.

"Right now, your blood sugar is probably 90. A healthy range for anyone, child or adult, is 80 to 120, so she is extraordinarily high," he said.

If we had gone home from the pediatrician's office without a diagnosis and Elle had eaten a normal breakfast, her body would have gone into something called *ketoacidotic shock*. She could have slipped into a coma, the doctor said. She would have been taken to the hospital by medevac instead of by car.

"A normal breakfast," Craig said. "So you mean to tell me that if she'd eaten a bowl of cereal this morning, she'd be..."

"Yes," the doctor said.

Fear shot through me. I was speechless. *How could our daughter be that sick without us knowing?* It was all I could do not to cry. I wanted to be strong for Elle, but my heart sank.

My God. What if I hadn't insisted on that urinalysis?

As a mother, I've often told myself I shouldn't push. I've always been a type A person, but I am sensitive about coming across as difficult. When faced with a problem, my first reaction is "Let's fix it!" I don't see the need to hem and haw about things. I'm also perfectly willing to do the work it takes to get what needs to be done, *done*. Yet there's a pressure I've felt as a mom to suppress that impulse every now and then. I try not to hover. I wouldn't want to jeopardize my kids' relationships with their friends or teachers or doctors or anyone else by seeming too "pushy." But at that moment, I was positive I would never doubt myself again when it comes to speaking up for the health and well-being of my children.

A nurse administered Elle's very first shot of insulin a few minutes later. "She's going to feel a lot better in about an hour," she told us.

In fact, Elle did feel much better within the hour. Her color came back. She fell asleep. I wondered why someone hadn't given her an insulin shot a whole lot earlier. Why did they make us wait?

Craig and I sat on the floor. The room was too small for anything other than the gurney where Elle now slept. There wasn't even a chair. So there we sat, mostly in silence, shell-shocked and scared.

It was sometime after midnight when Craig finally broke the silence.

"It's my fault," he said.

"What's your fault? What do you mean?"

"Diabetes is on my side of the family, Stefany, not yours," he said. He had tears in his eyes. "She got this from me."

"Don't. Don't do that. It's no one's *fault*, Craig," I told him. "There is nothing you could have done to prevent this."

I could tell that he didn't believe me.

What I didn't say out loud was what I was thinking: that *I* was the one who'd failed our little girl. I'm her mother. I should have done something sooner. I never should have let her get this sick.

As the hours stretched on, it became clear that we were not going to be moved into a regular room that night, so finally around 2:00 a.m. I turned to Craig and said, "You should go home." He didn't want to at first. "You can get our things. Get Elle her own pajamas so she's more comfortable. Check on the kids in the morning. Really, it's the best thing. I'm awake. I'll be here when she wakes up. I'm fine. Go."

I didn't see a doctor for the rest of the night. A nurse would come by now and then to check her vitals, but otherwise I sat there alone with my daughter, thinking about the person she was becoming.

Elle came into the world feetfirst—and, no, that's not a metaphor. She actually turned herself around before she was born and had to be delivered by C-section as a result. She loved musical theater more than anything, and she was already an avid performer who'd played in some regional stage productions. She even appeared in a local TV commercial—in which she wore a lab coat and played a young doctor. *How's that for a twist of fate*, I thought.

I didn't have a smartphone then. No one did. It was 2007. I had no way to look up answers to the million questions that flooded my mind. All I could do was sit there and look at my beautiful daughter and wonder, *If she really has this, if she's taking shots every day, will she be able to continue to do all the things she loves?*

I'm not a squeamish person. If I needed to give her shots, I could do it. I was sure I could do whatever needed to be done to keep her healthy, as long as someone told me what to do. But the fact that I'd gone from our pediatrician's office to a hospital to this ER without anyone giving me the information I needed to make her feel better was just about killing me. I felt helpless, and maybe a little hopeless—a feeling that was not familiar to me.

Elle woke up early the next morning absolutely starving. I took that as a positive sign. She looked good.

"How do you feel?" I asked her.

"Much better," she said. "Just *hungry.*"

I found a nurse and asked if it would be okay to give her something to eat. She told me that it should be fine. There wasn't any food service in the ER, so I wandered out to the Au Bon Pain in the lobby and grabbed some "healthy food" that I knew she'd like: a fruit cup, some cereal, and some yogurt.

Not forty-five minutes after eating that breakfast, Elle complained of a headache. Her color looked off again. She started moaning. She seemed nearly as sick

as when we'd first brought her in. I pushed the call button. I checked her monitors while we waited, trying
to make sense of the array of beeps and numbers and
symbols, and finally I saw that her blood glucose had
shot up to 500. I was horrified. I pushed the call button
again. Still, nobody came. Minutes ticked by. I pushed
the button again, blaming myself for making Elle feel
this way and remembering what the doctor said about
her slipping into a coma.

Still, no one came.

That's when I stepped out into the hallway—and
lost it.

"I am going to continue to speak with this loud
voice until someone gets me a doctor and comes to
talk to me!" I yelled. "We've been here for over twelve
hours, and we've only seen a doctor one time and my
daughter needs help. I don't know what I'm doing!"

I must've looked like a lunatic, standing there
screaming and disheveled in the clothes I'd been wearing for forty-eight hours. I'd endured plenty of sleepless
nights with each of my babies. I'd pulled all-nighters
all through school. I'd played Division I volleyball in
college. I prided myself on physical endurance. But the
mental and emotional fatigue had taken a toll. I was
irrational. I was angry. I didn't know what I needed to
do to keep my own daughter safe.

"Somebody needs to help me!"

Within thirty minutes of my *Terms of Endearment*

moment, they admitted Elle to the hospital and moved her into a proper room.

Later that day, after some more insulin, Elle felt good enough to take a walk. They told us there was a playroom with games and activities, so we headed down the hallway together. They'd placed us in a wing full of kids dealing with chronic illnesses, including kids living with cancer. We could see them through the open doorways, tied to dozens of tubes and monitors. Elle had never seen kids in that state before, and she definitely noticed the difference between her condition and theirs.

"I guess I don't need to be that scared," she said to me.

I felt thankful at that moment. I thanked God that we'd caught this. From what I'd seen and what I knew about diabetes, at least it was something we'd be able to handle. *This could be so much worse,* I thought. *Just look at Trent—he does great! He hasn't let diabetes slow him down. This is no big deal. Elle's tough. She can handle it. I can handle it. I'm sure I can.* What choice did we have, anyway?

Elle was already in great spirits. She seemed so much better after just a little bit of insulin that I really thought we were over the worst of it. Craig came back. We all laughed at the *Tom & Jerry* cartoons that were running and rerunning on TV. Eventually we met Dr. Alyne Ricker, a diminutive, gray-haired endocrinologist who examined and treated Elle. She was very much a clinician. Direct. No-nonsense. But she exuded confidence, and I appreciated that.

She pulled Craig and me aside for a parents-only meeting that afternoon, and I was sure we'd finally reached a point where we'd get our instructions, maybe an insulin prescription for Elle, and the go-ahead to take our daughter home.

"She's stable now," Dr. Ricker explained. "But we'll be keeping her here through the end of the week."

"What?" I said, shocked. "*Why?*"

"Because the next four days are about us teaching you everything you need to know to keep your daughter safe," she said, "and alive."

CHAPTER 2

Making Room

Dear Diary,

If you are worried about me, don't be. I'm fine. I'm feeling so good right now. There are a lot of scary things they had to do to me, but I was not scared. Well, I was scared at first, but now I am getting not scared anymore. I'm fine and people are supporting me and I feel so much better.

Love,

Elle, age 8

Mom, I thought I was crazy."

"What do you mean?" I asked.

Elle and I were alone again, waiting for discharge papers in her hospital room that Friday.

"Like, in math class," she said. "I couldn't sit there. I couldn't see. I felt horrible and sick and I didn't know why. But it wasn't all the time. Not like when you have a cold and you feel sick for a few days and then you start to feel better. I'd be sick and it would come on, like, right when I sat at my desk, and then sometimes I'd feel all better after math. Or after lunch, same thing. Those times when I was crying and you and Daddy asked me what was wrong and I didn't know. I mean, yeah, I thought I was crazy."

It was the first time I realized that this diagnosis offered some relief to my daughter. Knowing what's wrong, even if it's something difficult to hear, is certainly better than worrying that you're losing your mind.

During our weeklong crash course in diabetes education, we were able to figure out why Elle was suddenly doing so poorly in math. Her class was in the morning, about an hour after she ate breakfast. Her breakfasts were loaded with carbs, which meant her blood sugar was peaking almost exactly when math class was starting each day. She wasn't faking being difficult when she kept getting up to go to the bathroom or said she couldn't see the board. Her body wasn't making enough insulin to handle the carbs. Her vision was blurry because her system was saturated with sugar. She had to go to the bathroom because her body was trying to do anything it could to get rid of the excess sugar in her system. Her mood swings had nothing to do with a change in attitude. Everything traced back to the diabetes.

To avoid that in the future, we would have to monitor her constantly and do our best to keep her blood sugar under control. It would all be up to us.

The reality of that was just setting in when they sent us home.

The nurses handed us gigantic boxes full of supplies: test kits, books, brochures, prescriptions, syringes, glucagon kits for use in emergency situations only (like the EpiPens used by people with life-threatening allergies), posters showing the symptoms of high and low blood sugars that we were to hang on our walls and share with Elle's school, dozens of little glass vials of insulin that we needed to keep in our refrigerator, and more. They suggested we keep everything in one place. "The easiest place is usually the kitchen," they said.

We put the insulin in the refrigerator as soon as we got home, but that night, I opened all of the cabinets in my kitchen and stood back, staring at them. They were full. All of them were full.

I didn't have room. For any of it.

I left those boxes in the hallway and walked away.

When we'd first arrived at Children's Hospital, all I'd thirsted for were answers, but during the last three days there it felt like we were trying to sip water from a fire hose. They pumped us full of more information than we ever wanted to know about type 1 diabetes, which isn't anything like what most people think of when they hear the term *diabetes*.

Type 1 is an autoimmune disease with no cure. Unlike type 2, which predominantly impacts adults and can be the result of lifestyle choices or obesity, type

1 is a chronic illness requiring constant management of insulin doses along with careful monitoring of blood sugar levels, physical activity, and diet.

As I learned from our new Certified Diabetes Educator (or "CDE"), insulin is produced by the pancreas to help turn food into energy. Every organ in our body requires that energy to function. So without insulin, you die.

For some unknown reason, our daughter's immune system started wiping out her insulin-producing cells. There was nothing any of us did that caused it. And there is no known way to stop it. That's just what happens with type 1. And once Elle's insulin-producing cells were gone, they'd be gone forever.

The reality was that Elle would have to take injections of synthetic insulin from that point forward in order to survive. Insulin doesn't come in a pill. Elle's everyday existence would now include lots of needles. And replenishing her body's supply with synthetic insulin was fraught with complexity. Essentially, we would have to play the part of Elle's pancreas.

Elle would have to test her blood sugar by pricking her finger with a needle eight to ten times a day. *Every* day. Before and after *every* meal. *Every* time she wanted a snack. *Every* time she went out to play or went swimming or went to dance class. Every night, too, because sometimes, especially in kids, blood sugar can drop in the middle of the night for seemingly no reason at all.

While there are variables you can see—food, activity, and so on—there are also all sorts of variables we can't see in a child's constantly growing and changing body that can affect the body's blood sugar.

For people without diabetes, as soon as we *think* about eating a cookie, the pancreas springs into action and produces insulin to break down the sugars in that food. It then tapers off insulin production and keeps everything in balance automatically. Using synthetic insulin doesn't offer the same benefit. It's up to the person with diabetes—or in this case her parents or other adult caretakers—to take a blood sample and run it through a blood-glucose meter to figure out the correct amount of insulin needed to cover the carbs in whatever snack or meal is about to be consumed. And all of that needs to be weighed against the child's anticipated activity levels, since running and playing naturally burns more carbs than sitting or sleeping.

It was too soon for Elle to take responsibility for pricking her own fingers and giving herself injections. She practiced in the hospital by putting a syringe into an orange. They gave her a teddy bear and rubber gloves and medical tape and a fake syringe filled with water to practice with, too. "Am I doing it right?" she'd ask in her cute little voice, sitting in her pink flowered pajamas on her hospital bed and cradling that stuffed bear like a precious baby. But her eight-year-old body required incredibly precise doses of insulin, delivered via special syringes with tiny needles. One half-unit too much or too little could have "serious consequences," the doctors told us. *That's* why no one gave her any insulin on her day of diagnosis until after they'd completed a whole battery of tests. The fact is, too much insulin could kill her quickly, and too little insulin could kill her slowly.

Elle could've practiced injecting her teddy bear for days, but there was no way I would let her inject herself with insulin after learning all of that.

Historically, type 1 was referred to as *juvenile diabetes* because so many young children lost their lives from its devastating effects. We now know that the disease can be diagnosed at any age—as it was with Elle's uncle Trent—and even with the advent of synthetic insulin, the impact of the disease is still staggering. People with diabetes are two to four times more likely than other people to develop heart disease. Between 60 and 70 percent of people with diabetes develop nervous system damage. Diabetics account for 44 percent of all new cases of kidney failure, and the disease is the leading cause of blindness in adults.

Craig and I tried to shield Elle from hearing about these long-term risks at that point. Our daughter did not need to carry around the weight of all the potential side effects caused by this disease. Even that word, *disease*, seemed like too much. We decided early on that in our home, diabetes would be a "condition."

We could already feel her carefree childhood slipping away as it was.

The doctors and nurses insisted that the best and really only way to fight the long-term risks of diabetes was to monitor Elle's blood sugar levels and do everything we could to keep her in a healthy range, consistently, as much as possible. She would require checkups, along with something called an A1C test every three months, just to see how she was doing.

Needles and blood never bothered me. I'm a woman who asked for a mirror during my C-section so I could watch the operation. To me, learning to check Elle's blood sugar and give her insulin injections was reminiscent of learning to change her diapers for the first time. It started out a little scary, but by the end of the first weekend I felt like a pro. Still, I don't think it's possible to ever get comfortable having to draw your own child's blood. And the thought that I could overdose my daughter on the very medication she now needed to survive terrified me.

I suddenly longed for days when the biggest risk of messing up literally just meant a mess.

Learning about insulin was just the beginning, though. Our endocrinologist-ordered educational crash course included endless talk of carbohydrate counting, including math that would require a calculator to anticipate how much insulin Elle would need for every cracker she ate. I would need to teach myself just how the fat content of pizza causes the high carbs per slice to burn off more slowly in the body, sometimes over many hours at a time, and how to adjust her insulin dosage accordingly. They taught us the importance of proteins and fiber in the breakdown of sugars and how drastically even a body without diabetes is affected by the combinations of foods we eat. It was confusing, and it quickly became clear that this diagnosis would change our entire approach to eating and preparing food for our family.

We also learned that Elle's insulin requirements would change depending on whether she was in dance class or gym class, or happened to have a cold, or if she experienced a growth spurt, so we'd have to adjust her doses continuously.

Insulin wasn't a cure. It was more like an extremely delicate life-support system that would require constant maintenance and attention multiple times per day in order to keep working.

It seemed almost ridiculous as Craig and I sat impatiently in a cold conference room trying to absorb it all. Just when we thought we'd grasped it, there seemed to be a new wrinkle, another layer of complexity. How can anyone process this much information? I wondered. They must be exaggerating for effect. It can't be *every* time she eats. Not *every* night. How can anyone live like that?

Elle was patient and kind to every nurse and doctor

we met throughout our stay at the hospital that week. She listened, and learned, and seemed eager to show us how brave she could be. I had no idea whether any of this stuff was sinking in for her, though. Did she understand that her life would never be the same again? I didn't truly understand it myself.

I didn't want to.

Craig went back and forth to the hospital all that week. I was able to take time off and stay at the hospital for the duration, and I was thankful for that. I was thankful for a lot of things. One of our coping mechanisms in the middle of the crisis was to count our blessings. We were fortunate to live so close to Boston Children's Hospital. We were blessed to have a strong family network who could step in to care for Annah, Caraline, and William and who came to visit us in Boston when they could. I don't know what we would have done had we lived someplace without that network of built-in support. I already felt guilty for asking so much of them and hoped we wouldn't need to lean on them again once we got home.

Home. Just the thought of being at home with diabetes terrified me.

The doctors insisted that Elle should resume her regular activities as soon as possible. It didn't make sense to me, but they said it was important for her to get up and around so we could begin the "trial-and-error" phase of figuring out her particular insulin needs. A lot would depend on her schedule of activities, which included dance classes, voice lessons, and very often theater rehearsals.

Elle missed the audition for a production of *The Little Mermaid* while we were in Boston. A part of me was hoping she would forget about it in the whirlwind of that week, but during our discharge, she spotted the date on the paperwork and remembered.

"I'll call them," I told her on the ride home from the hospital. "Maybe they can find a part for you."

"Mom, no. You can't just call them. That wouldn't be fair to all the other kids who auditioned," Elle said.

"Well, you have a legitimate explanation!" I said, trying to lighten her mood.

"It doesn't matter. I don't want special treatment."

"Well, look, the doctors said it's important for you to resume your normal activities. It is very likely that you would have been doing this show if you weren't in the hospital, right?"

"Yeah. I guess so," she said.

"I'll just ask if they can let you be part of the production. Even if they make you a part of the scenery. You can play the part of a sea anemone or a rock or something," I said, which made Elle laugh.

When she finally relented, I called the theater. They were happy to have her, and she was thrilled to go. Elle went to her first play rehearsal the day after we returned from the hospital—and it was all I could do to let her leave the house. On any other day I would have dropped her off and picked her up at the end, but I insisted on staying and keeping an eye on her the entire time. No one else's parents were hanging around, and I wanted to spare Elle the embarrassment, so I sat in the back of the theater and pretended to read a book.

That night at bedtime, Elle looked exhausted, but her younger brother and sisters took forever to go through their bedtime routines, which meant it took a while for me to get to her. With four kids, bedtime was always a struggle in our household, but Annah, Caraline, and William seemed to be acting out that weekend: refusing to brush their teeth, continuing to play instead of climbing under the covers. I suppose that was the price I paid for being away from them for so long. Kids have all sorts of ways of letting parents know when their needs are not being met. I felt guilty about it, but my absence was necessary that week. Elle needed me.

By the time Craig and I had tucked them all in, Elle had already pulled up her covers and started to doze off.

"Elle, we need to check," I told her, prompting a groan.

I pricked her finger and found that her blood sugar was dangerously low. I immediately blamed myself, of course. I wasn't sure if I'd underestimated the amount of activity that day, or given her too much insulin with dinner, or what, but I was sure I'd done something wrong.

"Whoa, Elle, you need to eat something."

"What? No. I already brushed my teeth," she said.

"Sorry, but you need to eat. Do you want apple juice? Some Skittles?"

"I'm tired," she said.

"Well, part of the reason you're feeling so tired, Elle, is because you're low. Come on. Let's have some juice."

"Fine. But do I have to brush my teeth again?"

No one told me how to handle that one. Should we have tested before she brushed her teeth? They told me to test in the middle of the night, too. If she eats or drinks in the middle of the night, am I just supposed to let her teeth rot?

"We'll see," I said.

I brought her some juice, which she reluctantly drank. She then promptly drifted off to sleep while I held her.

I didn't make her brush her teeth again. I needed to pick my battles.

"Is she okay?" Craig asked.

"She's really low," I told him.

"What else can we do?"

"I'll retest in a few minutes and see."

I checked again fifteen minutes later and she was back in range, but that low worried me. I was afraid we'd misjudged her activity levels that day and I was afraid she might go low again in her sleep. I knew Craig had an early morning the next day, so I told him to just go to bed and I'd continue to check on her. I'd planned to test her again at 1:00 a.m. anyway, so I decided to just stay awake and get some work done. When I tried to wake her up at 1:00, she was listless. Elle had always been a heavy sleeper, so I couldn't tell if she was just tired or in serious trouble. She barely moved and seemed unable to speak. I tested her blood sugar again and she was dangerously low. *Again.*

I had no button to press, no nurse I could run down the hall to find.

I tried to get her to chew some Skittles. In the hospital, we'd found that just five of those rainbow-colored candies were often enough to pull her blood sugar back up. It didn't work, so I squeezed some yogurt into her mouth and did my best to get her to swallow. I held her head in my hands, hoping to see some visible sign of improvement in between pricking her delicate fingers and desperately hoping for a normal reading. *Is she swallowing?* We had been told it was important to couple fast-acting sugar with something that has protein in it so it would stick longer and burn slower, so we decided on yogurt, but now I worried that the yogurt wasn't acting fast enough by itself. I decided to give her orange juice. I put a straw in her mouth and tickled her cheek a bit, and she drank—even in her still-sleeping state.

I kept thinking, *I'm just a mom! I'm not an endocrinologist! This is my eight-year-old daughter who just wants to live a normal life. She wants to sleep! We both need sleep!*

It was after 1:30 a.m. when I pricked her finger and found that she was back in range again. The question was whether or not it would last. So I continued to hold her, and sometime after 3:00 in the morning I pricked Elle's finger once again and found that she was still in range. Apparently the yogurt combined with the OJ had worked. I took that as a lesson. My heart finally stopped racing. I fell asleep with my baby in my arms, realizing that this was going to be harder than I ever imagined.

Elle made it through that night, and she would make it through the next and the next with me sleeping beside her, listening to her toss and turn, and watching her breathe, just like I'd done when she was first born. When I did sleep, I'd wake up in the wee hours in a full panic and immediately check her, sometimes dripping tiny droplets of her blood on the sheets. Sometimes she was okay. Sometimes she wasn't. She never once woke up on her own no matter how high or low her blood sugar was, and I worried about missing a low blood sugar. So every night, I kept myself awake until 1:00 a.m. to check her one last time, then set my alarm to check her again before the other kids got up. As a result, diabetes became the last thing I thought about before I fell asleep and the first thing I thought about when I woke up every morning.

I kept telling myself it would get easier. Our pediatrician had promised that it would, so I tried to hold on to that hope. I kept telling myself that we were still in the trial-and-error phase and that once we were through the learning curve, we'd be okay.

Meanwhile, life went on. We didn't live in a vacuum. We had four children to take care of, and Craig and I needed to put on a brave face for them, too, because somehow this all had to fold into the frenetic daily regimen of our family of six. School. Lunches. Pickups. Drop-offs. Classes. Sports. Rehearsals. Dinners.

The dinners were especially trying. Craig had always been the chef in our household, often inventing and creating dishes as he went along. He rarely followed recipes, and yet somehow nearly everything came out tasting delicious. During Craig's early childhood, his mom was single and busy working and raising three boys, so he'd learned to cook at an early age. Later, to save money for college, he worked at a seasonal restaurant in the lakeside town where he grew up. The chaotic nature of restaurant work was great preparation for parenthood, he liked to say, and I always felt lucky to have married a man who could cook, because my own culinary skills were sorely lacking.

I wondered now if the need for precision in managing Elle's diet would change Craig's methods and style in the kitchen, or our enjoyment at the table. That very first weekend home, we had to make room for food scales, a slew of measuring cups, and a calculator on our countertop. Craig began learning what substitutions to make—brown rice instead of white rice, for instance—and we'd both have to learn how to go about shopping with glucose management on top of the priority list. In the long run, we were assured it would be better for our whole family to eat meals with more protein and fewer complex carbohydrates and to choose snacks with fewer added sugars. Of course, that would mean breaking some long-established eating habits.

I wasn't one of those moms who reads every label when shopping for my kids. In fact, I'm hesitant to admit this, but I had never read nutrition labels, ever. When we met with the registered dietitian at Children's Hospital, it felt like she was speaking a different language. Craig did most of our grocery shopping as it was, so the idea of trying to redefine how we shopped was just baffling to me.

Thankfully, Trent offered to help. He came to visit us in the hospital and promised to take us shopping as soon as we got home, so we could get Elle some "free snacks," whatever that meant.

A few days after we returned from the hospital, we met Trent at the grocery store to continue our education.

"First of all, shop the perimeter," he said. "The stuff that's going to give you trouble is all located in the middle of the store."

I'd never noticed, but all of the fresh fruits and vegetables, the dairy products, the meats, basically all the foods that make managing diabetes easier—and the foods that are generally better for you anyway—are located around the perimeter of the average grocery store. Apparently that's also where most of the "free" foods were located. Foods like cucumbers, or pickles, or celery, or cashews are considered "free" because Elle could eat them without having to take insulin.

Meanwhile, in the cookie and cracker aisle, Trent showed us the label on some fudge-stripe cookies and noted that the nutrition information was based on a 2,000-calorie diet. "Elle doesn't eat two thousand calories a day, so whatever you see here will have to be adjusted to her actual caloric intake," Trent advised. He also pointed out the serving size and just how different an actual serving size might be from what was on the label. That would require calculations, too. I was exhausted by the time we left.

After loading the groceries into the car, and just as Craig started the engine and Elle climbed into the backseat, Trent gave me a hug.

"How are you holding up?" he asked.

"Okay, I guess."

"I'm sorry I lost it at the hospital that day," he said. "I just kept thinking, I know what this diagnosis has meant for me, and I can't imagine what it's going to mean for Elle, and for you and Craig."

I choked up.

"I don't think I can have this conversation right now," I said. "I don't want Elle to see me get upset, okay?"

Trent nodded.

⸎

Back at the house, as we unloaded our stash of diabetes-friendly food, Craig tripped over one of the big boxes of diabetes supplies that I'd left in the hallway. He spilled a bag of groceries all over the floor.

"Why are these still here?" he yelled.

"Because there isn't any room," I said.

"Then we need to make room, Stefany!"

"When have I had the time? Huh?"

"Then I'll do it," he said.

"I need to do it, and I'll get to it when I can!"

"Well, can you get to it soon before somebody breaks an ankle?" he said.

I spotted Elle trying to make herself invisible as she scooted past us and ran up to her room. Craig spotted her, too, looked at me, then walked outside and slammed the door behind him.

It was all too much. We were frayed.

Elle needed to get back to school. I needed to get back to work. We couldn't stay in this all-consuming state of chaos any longer. We needed to get this "trial-and-error" stuff behind us and find some sense of normalcy. Soon.

CHAPTER 3

Work

"I have been raised to believe that anything is possible with hard work and determination."

—Elle, age 14

I did it. I went back to work. My boss agreed to let me start off just three days a week and to come in later than usual. I devised a plan to drop the kids off at their various schools, then work at home for a couple of hours, then go to Elle's school at 10:30 a.m. to check her blood sugar and administer a dose of insulin that would cover whatever she expected to eat at lunchtime. Then I'd make my commute—worrying about her the whole time we were separated, so much so that I'd find it difficult to concentrate at my desk.

After lunch, the school nurse would be responsible

for checking her, but the nurse was nervous about doing it and I think that made Elle nervous, too.

"Mom, it's so annoying," Elle told me. "She asks me so many questions! I don't want to have to tell her every single thing I ate, and how hard I played at recess, and everything like that. I only want to have those conversations with *you*."

I told Elle that it would get easier once the nurse got more comfortable. After all, we'd gone through an intensive training period at Boston Children's Hospital. The nurse was still adjusting. Honestly, though, I questioned how the nurse would handle the situation if anything went wrong. It worried me because she flat-out told me that she wasn't comfortable dealing with needles and injections.

Elle was annoyed at the constant interruptions in her day. Going to the nurse's office every time she needed to check was disruptive. After lunch. After recess. Before and after gym glass. She wanted to be compliant and follow every instruction to the letter, not only to keep her father and me happy, but also because she knew how much better she felt when her blood sugar was in range. She now recognized how sick she felt when she was out of range, and she wanted to avoid that at all costs. Still, it was hard for her.

Even with the added complexities and frustrations that came with diabetes, Elle seemed happy to be back in school. After all we'd been through, I honestly think the thing she craved most was routine. I know that's what I craved. I just wanted a Monday to be a Monday again, and somehow going back to work, even with the worry, even with these new routines, felt good.

Plus, I needed to get back to earning a living.

Thanks in part to Craig's support and willingness to help juggle work and the kids, I had managed to get through grad school at Harvard's John F. Kennedy School of Government just a couple of years before all of this began. We did it while raising three little girls under age six. I was pregnant with our youngest, William, during the final nine months of the program, and as graduation drew near, I could no longer fit my burgeoning belly behind the classroom desks. I had to sit sideways when I took my final exams. I'm not sure how we did it all, but somehow we made it work.

The sense of accomplishment was huge. I cradled newborn William in my arms as I posed for pictures in my cap and gown. I topped it all off by landing a dream job right there at Harvard after I graduated, working as a researcher for my favorite professor at the Business School, with expertise in crisis management, leadership, corporate social responsibility, and other areas.

Commuting to Cambridge most days took a solid hour and fifteen minutes when there wasn't traffic. And when is there no traffic in and around Boston? But my job wasn't a choice. We needed that paycheck. We needed insurance. With four mouths to feed, there was no way we could make it on one income. People may find that a little surprising given my family name, but it's true.

The Shaheens are bootstrap people. My father, William Shaheen, is the son of an immigrant family who settled in Dover, New Hampshire. He was the first person in his family to graduate from college, thanks in part to the Reserve Officers' Training Corps (ROTC) program. After serving as an army captain, he put himself through law school with help from the GI Bill. A few years later, President Carter appointed him to be the U.S. Attorney for New Hampshire. He served as a judge in our small town while I was growing up, and he still works as an attorney and businessman.

My mother, Jeanne Shaheen, was equally as passionate and hardworking. She started getting involved in public service by volunteering on presidential campaigns. New Hampshire is home to the first-in-the-nation primary every four years, and for decades she worked tirelessly in the trenches of long, grueling campaigns before she ran for office herself. She would eventually become a three-term governor, and in 2008 she became the first and only woman in U.S. history to serve as both a governor and a U.S. senator.

My parents taught my sisters and me the value of hard work, and we are incredibly fortunate to have grown up in such a big and loving family in New Hampshire—the best state in the nation. But my parents' success didn't make me independently wealthy. Hard work isn't an option. It's a necessity.

Craig and I both believe that downtime is a necessity, too, and we were anxious to do something fun with the whole family as soon as we could. So on Saturday, a week and a day after we brought Elle home, we piled into the minivan and trekked up to Maine for a visit to the Portland Children's Museum.

Craig would much rather have done something outdoors, but it was just too cold. Plus, this was our first family outing since the diagnosis, and I couldn't wrap my head around how we would care for Elle outdoors in the cold just yet. At a museum, at least I knew there would be a snack bar and bathrooms.

As it turned out, I struggled to figure out everything we'd need to bring with us. I must've made five trips back and forth from the house to the car, gathering snacks and test strips and a backup glucagon kit for Elle, in addition to William's blankie, and diaper bag, and stroller, and all of the usual little-kid paraphernalia.

After the coats and boots and hats and mittens were all stashed away at the museum's entry, the kids started pulling on me, raring to go—but I had to make everyone wait. Elle needed to check, and I could instantly see how uncomfortable she was being the one to blame for holding her siblings back from their fun.

The *snap* of the spring-loaded lancet Elle used to draw blood seemed to catch Caraline by surprise.

"Does that hurt?" she asked.

"Not really. I'm pretty used to it now," Elle said. "You want to try it?"

"No!" Caraline responded.

At lunchtime the kids had to wait while we checked her again. They were good. They were patient. But when I pulled up the back of Elle's shirt to administer an insulin injection in her lower back in the middle of the crowded cafeteria, Annah got quite the look on her face.

"Are you okay doing that in front of everybody?" she asked her sister.

"Well, what choice do I have?" Elle said.

All of this was new. All of it was challenging. It hadn't occurred to me just how blissfully unaware the little ones had been until that day. The tests and shots had happened mostly out of sight. They were six, four, and two. Their focus was elsewhere, until it wasn't. It was Craig and I who were left to sort out how to get William into a high chair and pour Annah some water and help Caraline in the bathroom at the same time Elle needed her insulin. This was our new normal now, whether we liked it or not.

We were just starting to adjust to it all when one morning the following week, Elle called me from school as I was rushing out the door. "Mommy, I don't feel good."

"What do you mean? Where's the nurse?"

"I can't find her," she said. She sounded awful. "She's not here. I don't know what to do. I'm scared."

I jumped in my car and drove like a maniac straight to Elle's school. The nurse made her way back to her office just as I arrived. Elle was nearly unconscious. Her blood sugar was extremely low. She was white as a ghost and sweating profusely.

"I'm sorry, Mommy," she whispered. "I don't know what I did wrong."

"No, no, Elle. You didn't do anything wrong. I'm so glad you called me," I said, relieved that she caught me before I left for Cambridge. What would have happened had I not been home?

That's when a new reality hit, and hit hard: There was no way I could continue to work sixty miles away from her. Craig was working in commercial real estate then. His job was unpredictable and often kept him away from the Seacoast, too. I could never live with myself if something happened to our daughter because I was too far away to keep her safe. I loved my job at Harvard, but in that moment, I knew that job was all but finished. I would have to find some sort of work closer to home.

Diabetes had already altered life as we knew it in my family. Now it was forcing me out of my job.

Craig and I had vowed to do whatever we could to make sure Elle continued living a "normal" life, but we quickly learned there is no "normal" in the life of a third-grade girl with diabetes. And the fact that we were forced to figure all of this out in the weeks between Thanksgiving and Christmas made it especially difficult. The holiday season is a stressful time for all families. Now, on top of everything else, each day brought new challenges, and new reasons for swings in her blood sugar levels. Going to the holiday book fair forced us to decide what to do when she wanted to eat a candy cane like all the other kids. Should we just say no? Or should we give her some insulin and risk a high blood sugar so she wouldn't miss out on a common holiday activity? For the most part, Elle was flexible. She was generally back to being the same old ready-to-please girl she'd always been. But knowing that we had to make these decisions, and that she had to stop and think about it when none of the other kids did, was tough.

"How much insulin does she need for that?" Craig would ask me as we tried to enjoy some sugar cookies while decorating the Christmas tree. Then we'd both look up the carbs and get the calculator to figure it out. Going to play at a friend's house meant talking to the parents to make sure they were willing to handle the added responsibility, and then figuring out what snacks to send with her. Then we'd get it wrong. I'd send her to ballet class with a big snack and a tiny dose of insulin, only to find that she'd come home pasty and miserable with a high blood sugar because apparently working on the bar didn't burn a ton of energy. Jazz class, on the other hand, sent her crashing to a dangerous low that required less insulin and more sugar.

Keeping track of all of her supplies was also a challenge. The school would call to say they were out of alcohol swabs or test strips or that they were having trouble with the backup meter we'd given them to check her blood sugar. So I'd drive over with replacement supplies or to provide additional instructions to make sure she could participate in a new gym activity or attend an off-site field trip.

I spent countless hours in the drugstore trying to sort out her prescriptions. Inevitably the insurance company wouldn't cover the type of test strips the doctor prescribed or the kind of insulin she needed and I'd have to spend hours on the phone trying to get the issue resolved. My favorite was when the doctor told us she should test six to eight times per day, but the insurance company only wanted to cover four test strips per day.

The headaches and responsibilities seemed to grow heavier as time went on—not lighter.

We kept telling Elle that her diabetes wouldn't keep her from doing the things that she loved, but Craig and I were twisting ourselves into knots trying to live up to that promise.

This cannot be as hard as it seems, I thought. *It's 2007, for crying out loud! There has got to be something out there that can make this easier.*

CHAPTER 4

Trials and Errors

"Diabetes has affected my life more than it should have...all the trips to the doctor's office and poking my fingers with a needle. It's been hard."

—Elle, age 10

Sometimes hope pops up when you least expect it.

I was feeling pretty hopeless the first time I left Elle at home for a night out. Weeks had gone by and it was still a struggle to get her safely through each day, but I'd long been scheduled to attend a political event with my mother, and with Craig's encouragement—and hers—I decided to go ahead.

Presidential election years in New Hampshire make for fascinating times. I stood in a room that night with some of the biggest political heavyweights in the country, surrounded by national media figures, and I couldn't tell you what any one of them said or did that entire evening. My thoughts were with Elle and the guilt I felt for leaving Craig alone with the responsibility that had weighed so heavily on our shoulders every day since her diagnosis.

Then something happened that made me feel like I was in the right place, at the right time. Dean Kamen, a preeminent engineer who is often described as the Albert Einstein of our time, pulled me aside. Dean invented the first insulin pump for people living with diabetes. We were hopeful that Elle would be able to start using an insulin pump in the coming year. From heart stents to dialysis machines to the Segway to clean-water filter systems for third-world countries, Dean Kamen's inventions and innovations have changed lives for the better all over the world. I'd been fortunate enough to work with Dean during my time at Harvard, and he'd known my mother and father for many years.

"Your mom told me about your daughter's diagnosis," he said. The man had tears in his eyes, and as soon as he said those words, so did I. "I'm so sorry."

"I know it doesn't help you right now," he continued, "but of all the chronic illnesses a child could be diagnosed with, diabetes is the best one." I had no idea what he meant by that, but he quickly explained. "There's so much cutting-edge research going on in the field, from drug therapies to the artificial pancreas, any one of which could change your daughter's life for the better in the next decade. We're so close, on so many fronts. There's real reason to hope. Okay?"

It occurred to me in that moment what a gift it was to have that man standing right in front of me. I felt very, very lucky, and I decided to ask his advice about something.

During our week at Children's Hospital, we'd learned about dozens of cutting-edge diabetes-related medical trials, any number of which Elle might be eligible to join.

Yale-New Haven Hospital was in the middle of a trial investigating a potential drug therapy aimed at extending natural insulin production in people living with type 1. Of all the potential studies my daughter could take part in, that one seemed the most promising and one that could actually improve her life. I'd read up on everything, but I wasn't sure it was the right thing to do. It seemed like a very scary proposition to let my baby be used as a guinea pig. So I asked Dean all about it.

"I know about that study. It's a good drug. The initial tests are so promising," he said.

"So this could really be good for her?" I asked.

"It could. And good for the cause, too. They need more pediatric patients in the trial before the results can be presented to the FDA," he said. "But no matter what you choose to do, just know that there's reason to hope. Very real reason to hope. Okay?"

These were not the encouraging words of a friend or relative who had read a few articles and was just trying to make me feel better. These words came from the mouth of a man with extensive knowledge about diabetes, science, and technology. He gave me hope. For the first time in weeks, I walked back into my home that night with something to think about that extended beyond the next time I'd have to prick my daughter's finger.

The medical trial that initially scared me now sounded like a compelling option. The catch was that Elle had to undergo some additional testing before we would know if she was eligible to enroll, and testing had to be completed within twenty-eight days of her initial diagnosis. Time was running out.

Craig and I talked about it and we agreed that it seemed like a very good thing to do, but the final decision wasn't up to us. It was Elle's body, and ultimately Elle's decision. Elle was the one who would have to be pulled out of school again. She was the one who would have to be put into another hospital and poked and prodded. I agonized over how to ask an eight-year-old to wrestle with such a difficult choice.

The idea that this medication could extend her body's ability to make insulin would surely make life easier. The very idea of it gave me hope. Finally, with just a couple of days to spare to get her enrolled, we sat Elle down to talk. She kicked her little legs back and forth, anxious to return to a dance routine she was practicing with her sisters, but she was wide-eyed and full of attention as we talked about the possibility. She seemed to take it all in, the pros and cons, the risks, the reminders about hospital gowns and needles and tubes.

Then she looked at us and said, "Sign me up!"

"Really?" Craig said.

"When can you sign me up?" she replied.

"Are you sure?" I asked.

"Absolutely," she said.

"It will mean two weeks in a hospital, and missing school and missing dance, and—"

"Mommy, if there's a chance this can help me, I want to take that chance. And if this medicine they're testing could help other people not get diabetes, or—"

"I don't think it will keep people from getting diabetes, Elle, but—"

"Or if it will help other kids to not have to get as many shots, then of course I want to do it. Why wouldn't I want to do it? There has to be something good that comes out of this, right?"

I was awestruck by her desire to help, but I also knew she was too young to fully grasp the trade-offs and ramifications of that decision. I still thought it was the right decision, though, so the next day I called the team at Yale-New Haven and started the application process.

⌒∞⌒

Saying yes to that medical trial marked the start of a series of new journeys for Elle and me. First of all, it sent us to New Haven, where we would be fully immersed in nothing but Elle's health for two weeks. I would stay with her full-time for the first seven days and then alternate with Craig, staying at a college friend's house near the hospital during the second week, when Elle wouldn't have to be confined to a bed but would need to stay close to the hospital. That meant saying good-bye to Annah, Caraline, and William again, and once again leaning on our extended friends and family for help.

"Mommy, you need to give me seven kisses 'cause you're going to be gone for seven days," Annah said as Elle and I gathered up the last of our things. Then Caraline hopped into my arms for a big hug and wouldn't let go. Caraline always seemed to need the most from me. She was the baby who fought taking a bottle when I had to go back to work and the one who had the hardest time saying good-bye at preschool drop-off. I carried her all the way to the door, and she started crying. My cousin had to pull her from my arms as she kicked and screamed.

Elle watched it all, silently.

As difficult as it was to reconcile that choice to leave the rest of my family behind, I was positive this trial was the right thing to do. I would deal with the guilt and fallout from the separation later.

Being confined in a hospital with my oldest daughter was a reprieve. It felt good to be able to focus on nothing but Elle and her needs for a while, free from school schedules and laundry and feeding four kids, and with the additional backup of a team of doctors and nurses. It was also just plain fun to bond with my daughter. We played board games, and worked on her homework together, and embarked on a romantic-comedy VHS movie marathon. (Yes, the hospital still had a dated VCR in the room.) It started to feel as if Jennifer Lopez, Julia Roberts, and Meg Ryan were our friends, and in the end, we decided that *You've Got Mail* was our favorite.

These types of trials rarely have enough volunteers, and it's easy to understand why. While it definitely helped us, it was a big commitment. Just the time away from work and the distance would make it impossible for so many.

Elle bonded with a nurse named Melissa, who was in her mid-twenties and also living with type 1. It was fun for me to see their relationship develop. Melissa took time to help Elle learn how to check her blood sugar all by herself. She taught her the importance of rotating and using both hands so her little fingers wouldn't get calloused. She even taught her how to properly measure and inject insulin herself. It was still too scary for me to let her administer insulin without adult supervision, but learning to give herself a shot was a huge step forward. Having the confidence that she could do it lifted her spirits immensely. So did some of the answers they gave her to the questions she had, including whether she had done something that may have caused her to get diabetes. "No," one doctor assured her. "You could've eaten birthday cake for every meal of your entire eight years of life and that wouldn't have caused you to get diabetes. It wasn't your fault."

It felt like a much-needed diabetes boot camp. For both of us.

I know for me, seeing all of those professionals working together to improve care for patients gave me hope. Not just hope for the future—that someday, perhaps within my daughter's lifetime, there might be a cure for this awful disease—but hope that Elle could survive and thrive with type 1 despite how difficult it all was every day.

I hoped Elle absorbed that message, too.

Being away from the daily pressures of home also gave me a chance to concentrate on learning everything I could about counting carbs and calculating insulin doses. In the beginning, I didn't know what I didn't know. Now? After being home with Elle? I realized what Trent was trying to tell us when he took us to the grocery store and explained that just because a label says a serving has 20 g of carbs, there is always more to the story. I needed to understand how to balance out the fats and proteins she'd be eating with those carbs in order to make better estimates and keep her blood sugar in check. These people had answers for me.

Those two weeks also solidified just how interested my daughter was in making something positive come out of her own struggles. The Shaheens had always been an activist family. We got involved. That's just what we did. We didn't turn a blind eye to the problems in our society or in our community. Craig, an advocate for the working poor, was that way, too. Seeing Elle's resolve made it perfectly clear that our new reality would turn into a very personal crusade. It was time for us to get to work so that one day Elle and millions of others living with diabetes would have a better quality of life and ultimately a cure.

I suppose I'd been molded to work for causes I believed in from the start. I remember "working" as a small child in political-campaign headquarters with my mom, sitting at a card table with a stack of three-by-five cards, truly believing that I was phone banking on my plastic Fisher-Price phone. I also vividly remember the moment when George H. W. Bush won the presidency in November 1988. My parents, who are both Democrats, were watching the results in our living room, and they were so disappointed by the news. They'd been upset with the outcome of presidential elections for most of my life at that point. I walked

into the living room and said to them, "I don't understand why you do this. Why do you work so hard when
you know you're going to lose?"

"There are things worth fighting for, even if you're
not going to win," my mom said to me.

"But why?" I asked. I truly didn't understand.

"Because what we're fighting for is bigger than
winning or losing at any one time," my dad explained.
"It's about making a difference for people."

I took their lessons to heart time and time again.
I always had. I remember in third grade there was a
school dress code that forbade the wearing of clogs. I
got clogs for Christmas—believe it or not they were
fashionable for a time back then—and I thought the
dress code was unfair. So I petitioned to get it changed,
and I won. In middle school I spoke out against pro-
posed cuts to the sports and music program budgets
during a public school board meeting. In college I
worked at a domestic violence shelter, advocating for
legal protection for victims, and shortly after Craig and
I got married, I started working as an advocate for early
childhood education. Later, after my girls were born,
I was part of a state agency tasked with improving
conditions for women inmates in New Hampshire—
revamping an outdated system that in this modern day
had removed computers from the women's prison and
replaced them with, of all things, sewing machines.

Advocating for anything that could improve the

lives of people with this disease, including my daughter, only made sense. It felt comfortably familiar to me.

As soon as we got home, I reached out to JDRF (formerly known as the Juvenile Diabetes Research Foundation). I offered to help in any way I could. That organization had been there for us from the start.

I remembered sitting on top of a heater near a window in Elle's room at Children's Hospital, desperate to take a shower and to sleep in my own bed, holding a blue backpack that someone from the hospital staff had given to us that day. Inside was a teddy bear and several books and DVDs about living with type 1. The backpack was from JDRF, and they called it the "Bag of Hope."

That backpack became somewhat of a symbol for me—a metaphor for what it would take to make lemonade out of the lemons we'd been handed. I realized that a backpack would simply be far too heavy to carry if it was full of the lemons of resentment and bitterness and self-pity. I couldn't burden my first child with the weight of that negativity.

Instead, we had to fill that backpack with the sweetness of hope and possibility and the opportunity to make a difference. That's just how I was wired, and JDRF seemed like a great place to start.

I also started talking to my mom about what was going on with federal funding for diabetes research. She was gearing up for a heated election season and was running again for the U.S. Senate in 2008. Back in 2002, after serving three terms as governor, she ran against John E. Sununu for U.S. Senate and lost. One of the issues in that campaign was stem-cell research. Sununu's vote was one of four needed to overturn our then-president's veto of stem-cell research. If my mother had won that election, there's a chance that research would have continued. The really ironic part? During a 2002 campaign event, Al Gore said that the advances in stem-cell research could lead to a cure for diabetes within ten years. Ten years! I had campaigned with my mom on that very issue, never knowing or imagining that my own daughter might someday need the promise of that research to hold on to hope. Now here we were, six years later, sitting in a research hospital surrounded by doctors and nurses who were as sickened as we were by the loss of all those years of research. It hurt to imagine how much closer we would be to finding a cure and to wonder how much more needless suffering would be endured because of the decision to essentially halt stem-cell research.

If stem-cell research had been funded and continued during those six years, there may well have been a cure or a significant new treatment on the way before my daughter was ten years old. Joining a fight to make sure that research moved forward faster than ever now seemed like the absolute right and necessary thing to do.

At this age, I know myself well enough to know

that I am happier when I'm on a mission. Following my daughter's lead in the fight for diabetes research and awareness lit a new fire in me like no other.

∽

Unfortunately, going through that medical trial didn't "fix" anything in our day-to-day life. It didn't eliminate or even reduce the daily and nightly challenges of Elle's condition. It didn't change the fact that we'd have to travel to Massachusetts to visit Dr. Ricker every few months for follow-up visits, not at Boston Children's Hospital but at Dr. Ricker's primary place of practice, Joslin Diabetes Center—one of the top diabetes research facilities in the world. It struck me how lucky we were to live in the Northeast, within driving distance of some of the greatest hospitals and doctors on Earth. I remember thinking, *What must it be like for families who don't have access to this kind of care?*

On our first follow-up visit with Dr. Ricker, I received a sharp reminder of how tough type 1 can be, even with the best possible care. Upon arrival, Elle had to go through a series of blood tests. She was a trouper, but it is never fun to have people poke needles into your arms and fingers. Eventually we wound up in Dr. Ricker's office with Elle sitting next to Dr. Ricker as she studied the results of those tests.

"Well," she said, "your A1C is better than it was

when you were first diagnosed, but still higher than we would like it to be."

"What?" Elle said. She looked worried. "Mom, what does that mean?"

I knew the answer. We'd heard about it in the hospital and I'd read more about it since. We'd shielded Elle from as much as we could, but she did need to know why this regular test was so important.

Dr. Ricker quickly explained in her matter-of-fact way that an A1C test showed the average range of Elle's blood glucose levels over the previous three-month period. The goal for a young person was an A1C reading between 7 and 7.5. The more we could keep Elle in that range, the better chance she had of avoiding the long-term effects of diabetes. Elle already knew that blindness was one of those long-term effects.

Elle looked horrified. "So what did I get?" she said, as if she were talking about a grade on a test at school.

"Your A1C is 8.3," Dr. Ricker said.

I could see the tears forming in Elle's eyes.

"Honey, it's okay. We're still learning. We just need to catch more highs and keep you from going low a little better, that's all," I said.

"Yes," Dr. Ricker said. "This is not too surprising given how recently you were diagnosed. I've seen far worse, believe me. Keep up your hard work and don't get discouraged. If you keep checking your insulin with every meal, you'll get there."

In the car, Elle was quiet. Then she asked me, "Mom, am I going blind?"

"No! Elle, no. There's no immediate danger from that A1C number, okay? It's just a measure of how you're doing overall. Like I said, we're still learning. We'll get it in range. We may just need to make some adjustments, but we'll get there."

"I don't want to go blind," she said.

"Elle, you're not going to go blind. We will never let that happen."

Deep down, I had no idea if I could actually make that promise. Especially since she was experiencing so many highs and lows that I couldn't figure out how to prevent.

A few days after that appointment, Elle and Annah got all bundled up to go out sledding with some kids from the neighborhood. We went through the standard parent-child checklist: hat, gloves, boots, socks, scarf, jacket, zipped and tucked so the cold couldn't get to their skin, and off they went. We'd tested Elle's blood sugar not long before the bundling process and she was in range. She'd had a good lunch. We live in a safe community. She and Annah were impatient to go meet their friends, and they wouldn't be too far ahead of me. I was juggling Caraline and William, who needed extra help to get bundled up, so I said, "Sure. Go ahead."

Ten minutes later, as I continued to wrestle with the little ones to get boots, hats, and mittens on, I noticed Elle's test kit sitting on the counter. She'd forgotten to bring it with her. Then I thought, *Did Elle remember to bring any sugar with her?*

I panicked. I left Craig to get Caraline and William bundled, grabbed the kit and a bag of Skittles, and ran out into the cold with my slippers on to find her. Skittles were Elle's go-to, fast-acting sugar of choice, and chances are she had a bag of them stashed in her jacket pocket. We'd learned to keep them in all sorts of at-the-ready places. I just needed to be sure.

When I found her a few minutes later, she was listless and sitting alone on the sledding hill.

I tested her as quickly as I could and found that her blood sugar had dropped below 60 in record time.

"I'm sorry. I'm so sorry," she cried.

"Elle, *I'm* sorry. You can't apologize. It's not your fault!"

"I'm sorry!" she continued. It was clear to me she wasn't just sorry for forgetting her test kit and Skittles. She was sorry that her fun had been interrupted. The rest of the kids were all yelling and laughing and having a blast on the hill. She was sorry that she suddenly felt so miserable. She was sorry for making me run out in the snow in my slippers.

I was the one who should have been sorry. I felt, once again, like I'd let her down.

Elle shoveled Skittles into her mouth ravenously and we waited the agonizing time it took for her blood sugar to climb back into range. What if I hadn't run after her? My daughter could have been minutes away from a seizure, all because I'd forgotten to remind her to take her test kit and a snack with her.

She was too weak to walk, so we sat there for nearly twenty minutes in the freezing cold before I could check her again and see if she was back in a safe range. She wasn't. She was still low, but her blood sugar had come up some, and we thought we'd better get her inside. So I helped her up, all cold and wet, and we waddled back toward the house.

"What happened?" Craig said, consoling our younger children and staring at my snow-covered feet.

"She's okay," I said. "It was my fault."

He grabbed a blanket and wrapped Elle up in a warm hug, giving me a look that was all too reminiscent of the look he'd given me back at the Christmas-tree farm.

Searching for answers as to what might have caused such a sudden drop, I called our CDE at Joslin. She explained that the body works hard to stay warm when it's cold, so low blood sugars are common when playing outside in cold weather. That never would have occurred to me. I still had so much to learn.

From then on, I had to take into account the temperature outside each time Elle went out to play. I also vowed it would be the last time I ever let Elle walk out of the house without going through an entirely new parent-child checklist. "Did you check? When did you check? Did you take insulin? How much did you take? Do you have your test kit? Insulin? What do you have for snacks? Where are your Skittles? Are they in your backpack or your coat pocket? Please double-check. You can't leave without them."

To me, this rundown was essential. To her, I am sure it felt like nagging. But if nagging was the answer to keeping her safe, so be it. Let her and anyone else within earshot be annoyed. There are worse things I could be as a mother, I thought. The constancy of it would cause even *me* to grow annoyed at the sound of my voice at times, but I would never let my daughter leave our house again without answering those questions. To manage my own worry, I just had to ask.

Even with that new checklist, things would get missed or forgotten. The spring thaw and transition into summer were marred by dozens of additional near misses. The change in routines, the lack of predictable school-dictated lunchtimes during summer break, the adrenaline spikes from nerves before a theater performance, the play dates, the outings on the water and in swimming pools all brought new challenges to managing our daughter's condition. Craig and I continued to turn ourselves inside out to help her manage the variables, and each time we found our way through a new situation, it felt like a little victory. Yet with every new victory, new setbacks emerged—as if diabetes had an endless supply of reinforcements waiting in the wings.

By the time Elle started fourth grade that fall, she was given the option to use an insulin pump—a device she would wear on her waist that looked a little like one of those rectangular beepers from the late 1990s that were big enough to display messages. The pump carries insulin, which flows from a small chamber inside the device through tubing that is connected to a "site." The site is attached using a very daunting 9-mm needle, which threads a small catheter under the skin that would have to be changed every three days. After it was attached, we wouldn't have to inject her with insulin through a syringe six to eight times a day anymore, as we'd grown accustomed to doing. Instead, insulin would be infused into her body through the pump. That in and of itself felt like a huge relief to all of us.

The pump wasn't a very intelligent device. It had no way of knowing if the blood sugar was dropping or rising, and therefore didn't eliminate her need to test as frequently. It would be up to us, and to Elle, to tell the pump what to do. But it *would* give Elle some freedom from having to constantly go to the nurse's office for injections.

We packed her lunches every day with healthy foods low in added sugars and complex carbohydrates. I also included a sticky note with a list of the total carbs in the entire lunch, and then the number of carbs in each individual item, so that Elle could tell the pump how many carbs she was eating. We kept a copy of a book called *The CalorieKing* in our kitchen and a pocket-sized version in the car and in my bag wherever we went. It lists the carbs and calories of nearly every food imaginable, so I could look up a medium-sized apple and see that it has 15 grams of carbs, or a large carrot has 8 to 10 grams of carbs, and so forth. (I soon had all of the most-common foods memorized.) The pump would deliver the correct dose of insulin as long as we told it how many carbs Elle was eating.

But there were times when the site would fall off at school and I would have to drive in to help her reinsert it. There were also times in the life of a fourth-grade girl when it just wasn't convenient to walk around wearing a beeper-like device on her waist. Because it was tethered to her body and clipped to her belt or the waist of her pants, she had to work around it every time she went to the bathroom. It made costume changes more difficult during her theater performances. She hated the feeling and the heft of it during dance class. It was too heavy to hang on a nightgown, or her underwear, which made it awkward when going to bed. She was never to be unattached except when she took a shower, so there were all sorts of trade-offs. Still, overall, the pump did make the administering of insulin a little bit easier and a little less messy, and at that point even a little relief felt like a lot.

With the pump and a whole lot of day-to-day experience under our belts that fall, I started to feel like maybe this life full of knot-twisting effort wasn't so bad.

Elle landed a role in the musical *Schoolhouse Rock* at the Seacoast Repertory Theatre—a professional regional theater that happened to be located right in our city. We made it through the whirlwind schedule of evening rehearsals and multiple performances with the help of a supportive cast and crew who looked out for Elle and made sure she was okay. The stage manager even took the time to let me show him how to use glucagon—an emergency glucose injection for use in case of seizures brought on by extremely low blood sugar. Craig and I practiced with that big, thick-needled syringe at Boston Children's Hospital, stabbing it with massive force into an orange. The needle would have to be punched deep into Elle's thigh if she were ever having a seizure.

"Don't worry about bruising her," the nurse said when she showed us. "A bruise won't kill her."

It was scary. We kept those glucagon kits everywhere: in the kitchen, in the nightstand, in Elle's bright-yellow diabetes bag that she now carried with her wherever she went. I vowed that I'd watch over Elle closely enough that we'd never have to use one, and in fact we'd never had to use it even once that entire year. We had an emergency supply of glucose gel stashed in one of our kitchen cabinets, too, which we could squeeze into her mouth if she ever had a seizure and was unable to swallow. We'd gone nearly a whole year without needing to use any of that scary stuff.

It didn't often feel like it, but as I watched her tackle her theater endeavors, I realized that we were managing. Somehow, we were managing.

The onslaught of the holiday season and the most wonderful overeating time of year began with Halloween, of course. Based on everything we'd been through, and our months of doing everything we could to avoid junk food, Craig and I thought it would be a good idea to put apples out for the trick-or-treaters instead of leaving a big bowl full of candy on our stoop like we usually did while we walked around our neighborhood and, later, went to our neighbor's annual Halloween party.

"Dad! No!" Elle pleaded.

"Kids will think we're *horrible*," Annah begged him. "Please don't. It's embarrassing!"

"It's the right thing to do, and I'm doing it," Craig insisted, and I backed him up.

We got a lesson in what kids thought about receiving "healthy" snacks when a pack of adolescent boys started smashing our apples all over the sidewalk, just as we were getting ready to leave. Craig was carrying a big tray of lasagna when he spotted them and ran to the door—dressed in his full party costume as a samurai warrior. "Stop what you're doing right now and get out of here!" he yelled. I can only imagine the story those boys tell of one crazy lasagna-wielding samurai.

Elle and Annah witnessed the scene through the window and were mortified.

There wasn't a guidebook for us to follow. We were both trying to do the right thing, to set good examples, to make Elle feel as if she didn't have to miss out on the fun of the holiday season. Was letting her and all of the other kids eat candy the better choice? Who's to say, really? We certainly couldn't force every household in the neighborhood to hand out fruits, nuts, or stickers. And it seemed unfair to cut Elle off from the treats. We would just have to be extra vigilant in our testing and treating to try to keep her blood sugar in check. And that Halloween night we were, and she was fine.

All in all, our day-to-day life went pretty smoothly that fall. Elle went and auditioned for another show at Seacoast Rep and landed a lead role in *Meet Me in St. Louis*, which was set to open the day after Thanksgiving. I felt good knowing that diabetes wasn't stopping her from doing the things she loved and was overwhelmed by the notion that we were quickly approaching the one-year anniversary of her diagnosis.

It would be our first "diaversary"—the anniversary of Elle's diagnosis. A day we would never forget.

CHAPTER 5

Darkness

"I just wanted the show to go on. The show must go on."

—Elle, age 9

I suppose I could blame my mood that Thanksgiving on the shorter days and the colder temperatures, but as we all sat down for dinner that year, I wasn't feeling very thankful. The daily, yearlong battle to manage Elle's type 1 had left me angry and fed up.

I wanted our simpler, before-diabetes life back.

We'd decided to stay home that year in part because of mounting financial pressures, but also because I couldn't imagine packing up all of Elle's supplies and keeping track of everything in the strewn-about suitcase reality of a crowded hotel room with four kids. Plus, I had soured on our new tradition of Thanksgiving treks to the White Mountains. The idea of watching our children swim in that pool or go to that same Christmas tree farm where the signs of Elle's diabetes first emerged elicited far too many sad thoughts. Not to mention new fears. Everything I associated with Elle's diagnosis reminded me that Annah, Caraline, and William were also at risk. The siblings of a child with diabetes have a higher risk of developing the disease. Every year from now on, we would have to have all three of them tested for the genetic markers for diabetes. It would now be a part of their annual routine to trek down to Joslin Diabetes Center, to endure the drawing of blood and the wait to find out whether they, too, would one day suffer through the finger pricking, insulin shots, and their parents' constant worry.

I watched Elle like a hawk in the company of our extended family that afternoon. Thankfully it seemed as if we'd calculated her insulin correctly, despite the added complexity of that oversized meal at such an odd time. The only issue came before bedtime when I had difficulty getting Elle to eat a snack.

"Ugh, Mom. I'm just not hungry," she said.

"I know and I'm sorry, but I need you to try and eat something," I said emphatically. I kept bothering her until she finally conceded.

Elle needed to eat before bed in order to keep her blood sugar stable through the night. Every night. We'd learned that lesson the hard way in that first year. I lost count of how many times she'd tested low in the middle of the night and I'd had to wake her to eat or slip a straw into her mouth and tickle her cheek to get her to drink something.

She finally relented and ate a green apple with peanut butter before brushing her teeth and going to sleep. Without any insulin, that snack provided plenty of fiber and protein to carry her until morning. Not to mention, green apples and peanut butter had become one of Elle's favorites.

I tested her around 1:00 a.m. as always, and she tested perfectly in range. I went to bed—only to be woken by the sound of Craig's bloodcurdling scream.

"Elle!"

I had never heard a sound like that come from my husband in all of our years together. I bolted out of bed. It was light out. It was morning already. I was shocked. I glanced at the clock and saw it was just after 7:00 a.m. I threw on my robe and ran to the kitchen to find the floor covered in a sea of cashews, a kitchen stool knocked to the ground—and my daughter convulsing in my husband's arms. She was having a seizure. *Oh God, oh God, please don't let her die.* Craig lifted her quivering body and carried her to the couch in the living room as I picked up the phone and dialed 911. I opened the supply cabinet and pulled out a glucagon kit, rushing it into Craig's hands as the dispatcher picked up. "My daughter's having a seizure. A major seizure. We need an ambulance. She has type 1 diabetes. Please hurry."

The dispatcher told me an ambulance was on its way and to stay on the line. I was terrified. Craig's hands were shaking as he struggled with the syringe. We were both in a state of panic, desperately trying to remember how to use it.

"Do it, Craig," I pleaded.

Craig held that thick needle in his right hand and raised it high as Elle convulsed with her eyes open and her jaw clenched. He hesitated.

"Just do it," I said. "Hurry!" He plunged down hard on our baby's thigh, delivering the dose in one swift blow. It wasn't until he pulled it back out that we both realized we'd forgotten a step. The vial of powder needed to be mixed and dissolved in the liquid *before* it was injected. She hadn't received the actual medicine she needed—only a saline solution. The fear that we'd just made a deadly mistake stabbed us both so hard it took our breath away.

"Glucose gel," I said, hurrying to the kitchen. I couldn't find it. I pulled all the supplies out of the cabinets and it wasn't there. "I can't find it!" I yelled.

"Should we try another shot?" Craig yelled back.

I ran to my daughter with a carton of orange juice and tried pouring it into her clenched mouth, spilling juice everywhere and not helping her one tiny bit. We rolled her on her side. We held her. I held her tongue.

"Elle? Elle?!"

She didn't respond.

Just as we were about to grab another glucagon syringe, we heard the siren. Craig opened the front door. Two EMTs rushed in. I stepped back, helpless, and Craig held me as we watched those men put our daughter on a gurney. The EMTs managed to get a proper dose of glucagon into her system. Her convulsing finally stopped, and for a very long moment her stillness terrified me.

"She's stabilizing," one of the men said.

I finally took a breath. In a quivering voice, I asked Craig what happened.

"She came into the kitchen and tripped over the stool. I asked if she was okay, and she said, 'Yeah,' and then she opened the cabinet and took out the cashews. She didn't look too good, so I told her, 'Let's get you something with more sugar,' and she dropped the whole can. I said, 'You'd better sit down and check,' and she collapsed!"

"Okay," an EMT said. "We need to get her to the hospital. Does one of you want to ride with her?"

"Yes!" I said. I looked at Craig. Thankfully Caraline and Annah were at a sleepover at their cousins' house, and William slept right through the ordeal.

"Go," Craig said. "I'll come as soon as I can."

I ran upstairs and threw on some clothes. We followed the EMTs out to the street as they wheeled her outside. After they lifted her in, I climbed into the back of the ambulance. The doors slammed and we lurched forward, sirens wailing. A few minutes later, Elle opened her eyes.

"Can you tell me your name?" an EMT asked her. "What's your name?"

He asked multiple times with no answer.

Then, finally, Elle said, "Oh. I'm Elle Shaheen."

I started sobbing.

"Elle Shaheen? Elle Shaheen?" he said. He spoke with a tone of recognition that would typically be followed by a question about my mother. *Not now,* I thought.

"Are you the Elle Shaheen I just saw in *School House Rock* at the Seacoast Repertory Theatre?" the man asked.

"Yes!" Elle said. Her eyes opened widely now and her face lit up. I will never, ever forget the look on that precious little face of hers.

The two started talking about the theater. Elle was groggy as she explained to him that her new show was set to open that very night. He asked her all about it, and she seemed to answer everything clearly. I listened intently for signs of slurred speech or incoherence. There were none. We arrived at the hospital a few minutes later, and on the way into the emergency room, the EMT announced to everyone, "Hey, we've got an actress here who has a show to do tonight, so let's take good care of her and get her out of here, all right?"

I appreciated his warmth and optimism almost as much as I'd appreciated his getting my daughter safely to the hospital. Portsmouth really was the perfect place to raise our family. Still, I thought, there was no way Elle would be doing her show that night. She'd be devastated. *I hate diabetes. I hate it!*

Having a seizure is more exhausting and taxing on the body than running a marathon. Every muscle expends its energy reserves. According to everything I'd heard and read, Elle would likely sleep for most of the next twenty-four hours. So once it was clear that she was stable, I called the show's director to let him know what had happened. He insisted on holding out hope that Elle might feel better by that evening, but he also said he would call the whole cast in early to try running scenes without her. The theater was small, and so were its budgets. Elle had no understudy. I worried that without her, there would be a cloud over opening night.

After sleeping for an hour, Elle woke up and vomited.

"Mom, what time is it? I don't want to be late to the show," she said.

"Just relax, honey. Get some rest, okay?"

She promptly fell back to sleep. The doctors told us the vomiting was most likely an allergic reaction to the glucagon. She kept dozing off, waking up, and vomiting, again and again—asking about her show every time she opened her eyes.

The doctors decided they needed to rule out anything other than a diabetes-related seizure, which required a battery of tests, including a CAT scan. Craig joined me at the hospital as we waited for results. Everything came back normal, but the day seemed to drag on forever.

When Elle woke up around 4:00 p.m., she stayed awake for the first time without needing a bucket. She looked at the clock.

"Whoa! We've got to get out of here," she said. "I've got a show to do!"

It was stunning. Elle had no idea just how traumatic her day had been. She didn't see it from the outside. She'd been unconscious throughout the seizure and had slept through most of the tests.

"Elle, I just don't think it's possible. I know you're going to be disappointed," I said, "but they've called the cast together and they're going to rework the scenes you're in so the show can happen tonight without you. It will be okay. It's not your fault."

The doctor walked in as I was talking.

"Well, if she wants to do the performance, there's no reason she can't," he said.

How about the fact that my heart can't take it! My daughter was in a hospital gown. She'd been vomiting the entire day after suffering a major seizure. I wished he hadn't said anything. I looked at Craig in disbelief and he motioned for me to come into the hallway with him.

"If the doctor says it's okay, then it's going to be okay," he insisted.

I'm sure he was terrified, too, but in that moment I needed his calming presence. I was rattled. Maybe even more rattled than I'd been on this very day a year earlier.

Soon after the doctor's declaration, they let us go home, where Elle promptly fell asleep on the couch with her feet in my lap. It was just before six when she woke and sat right up. "Mom, I'm ready to do the show. I feel good. I feel good!"

The last thing I wanted to do was let her walk out of that house, but I looked in her eyes and simply had no choice. "Okay," I said, and off Elle went, bouncing into the bathroom to take a quick shower. I could not understand where she got her energy. We arrived late for her call time, but Elle still managed to dress in full costume and makeup long before the director yelled, "Places!" I handed the stage manager about a week's worth of Skittles to keep at the ready backstage.

Craig and I took our seats in the front row with three glucagon kits, some Gatorade, and yet another bag of Skittles all stuffed into my purse. I reached my hand into the bag to double-check that they were still there as the house lights went down, and suddenly it all washed over me. I tried to hold it in, but I couldn't. The music started and the stage lights came up and I caught my first glimpse of my daughter on that stage, and I started crying. Craig took my hand and gave it a squeeze, but I could not stop. I cried through the entire play—sitting in the darkness, watching her dance, blaming myself again and again for allowing her to suffer that seizure.

Elle saw me sobbing during her final bows and looked at me like, "*Mom!* What is your problem?"

It was the first time I fully recognized that I could try to do everything right and might still not be able to keep her safe. I went over everything a thousand times in my mind and I was positive I had done all the things I was supposed to do, and still this had happened. Despite everything I'd done to try to manage the situation, type 1 diabetes had proven to me that it could not and would not be "controlled."

I made Elle sleep in my bed that night.

"Mom, I'm fine. I can sleep in my own bed," she said.

I insisted.

Seeing my daughter suffer that seizure tore me up inside. It scarred me. How could I possibly be expected to accept that it could happen again, with no warning, at any time? Once again I found myself thinking, *It cannot be possible that people live like this in this day and age. There has to be a better way.*

I wondered whether it was this difficult for every young person living with type 1. One of the ER doctors asked whether Elle might have hypoglycemia unawareness, a condition that prevents the person from feeling when their blood sugar starts to drop—a condition that is difficult to diagnose. Yet another unknown.

We're human. We adapt. We find ways to manage the unpredictability of life. I had done that by believing I could control this, when in fact, all I could do as a parent was to anticipate and monitor her condition as best I could and then treat and react accordingly. Intellectually, I understood that distinction. Yet I suddenly felt as if I'd been living a lie. As if I'd been moving through the world pretending for an entire year. I had fooled myself into believing that if I was on top of it enough, in tune enough, educated enough, perceptive enough, attentive enough, that I could influence the outcome. That I truly had the power to keep her safe. All parents must do that to some degree. We convince ourselves that if we do all the right things, we can keep our children safe from harm. The reality, the devastating truth that crushed me that night, was the horrible realization that no matter what I did, harm could find her anyway.

CHAPTER 6

Pressing Paws

"My grandfather has this Popsicle Stick Theory that
if you have one leftover Popsicle stick, you can break
it easily. But when you have a lot together, it's hard
to break them. Each one of our stories is like strong
Popsicle sticks put together."

—Elle, age 9

I often think about how we got through our darkest
days. I suppose it's because we were fortunate enough
to be surrounded by family and friends whose love and
support carried us even before we had reason to hope
that things would get better.

My father, who is notorious for his perpetual sense
of optimism, just wanted to take the hurt away. He
would promise, "It will get better," doing his best to
reassure me through my tears. "You'll get through this.

We will get through this together," he'd say, and I listened and did my best to believe him, just as I did when I was a little girl with hurt feelings after being left out or finding a giant beetle in my bed. I wanted to believe him now because I *had* to believe that life could get better.

My mother would patiently listen to my frustrations over regular battles with our health insurance company and offer her own reassuring words. My sisters would call to check in on us often, too. Stacey, the middle of us three Shaheen girls, would offer to take Annah, Caraline, and William when we needed to bring Elle to appointments; and Molly, the youngest, always provided comic relief, giving me a chance to focus on something other than what was happening at home.

My cousins and aunts were a huge source of support, too, stepping in to help with the kids whenever we needed a hand, or a place for dinner, or a chance to cry. The Shaheen family stuck together, and sometimes just knowing that I could count on them made it easier to face the day.

My closest friends from childhood and my formative years provided me with my own private lifelines. I remember a conversation with one particular friend that helped pull me out of a dark place. I was feeling sorry for myself late one night after I finished cleaning the kitchen and was waiting to check Elle's blood sugar again. "I don't think I can do this anymore," I lamented. After listening intently and with love in her heart, she replied, "Yes, you *can*. What choice do you have? And frankly you don't have the energy to doubt yourself." What she understood and helped me to realize in that moment was that I did not have the capacity to resist or fight my reality. She forced me to hear myself and to realize that the heaviness of that voice in my head wasn't serving me well at all. I needed to find ways to silence it. I knew that things could be worse. After all, I still had my daughter. It was time to stop being angry that things were the way they were and focus on doing what I could to make life better.

Sometimes the fullness of life itself carried us through, too. As strange as it seems, "the witching hours," as Craig and I call them—those chaotic hours between after-school and bedtime filled with homework and dinner and baths and more—became a time of respite. Everything was so hectic during those hours that there wasn't time to dwell on the life-or-death struggles of Elle's diabetes. Instead, it was just another part of the day-to-day management of our lives.

As the kids grew, Craig started coaching Annah's volleyball team and working to channel William's baseball obsession, while Caraline gravitated toward the performing arts like Elle, and I ran those two to rehearsals and voice lessons and dance classes. With four kids, the divide-and-conquer of it all was necessary. I'm not sure how I wound up being the theater mom. I was a sports kid growing up. In fact, Craig had been the assistant coach to my volleyball team way back in high school, where we'd first met. I suppose the day-to-day management of diabetes made it more practical for me to be the primary juggler of Elle's activities, and yet we all served as cheerleaders and spectators at each other's games and events whenever possible.

No matter how busy all of that became, the kids needed food, and bathing, and bedtime stories, and tickle fights before lights-out. And even with all the difficulties we faced, there was laughter. The silliness of childhood emerged in Caraline's jokes, and one of the girls would inevitably plug in an iPod after dinner, so the whole family would wind up dancing to the Jonas Brothers or Beyoncé while we picked up the dishes.

Days go by. Time passes. Some things get better, even while other things get worse.

I began to look at life in two parts: BD and AD, "before diabetes" and "after diabetes." And there is no doubt that a big part of Elle's happiness (and my sanity) in our AD life sprung from an ever-growing passion to raise awareness, participate in research, and join in the fight to find a cure for diabetes. Focusing on making life better for others helped both of us to focus less on how difficult life was for her. The work was replenishing—even though at times it was frustrating.

One of the biggest challenges to advancing new treatments and technologies in the fight against diabetes is the difficult regulatory climate in Washington. FDA restrictions make it extraordinarily arduous for new technologies, especially medical devices, to make their way to the marketplace. And for far too long, researchers in the field who rely on federal funds have been stymied in their search for both treatments and a cure by that broad, misguided ban on stem-cell research. The more we learned, the more motivated we grew.

Stem cells are the building blocks of just about everything in our bodies—and stem-cell research holds tremendous promise for curing a wide spectrum of human ailments, from diabetes to Parkinson's disease to spinal cord injuries. Working to overturn that ban was something my family had done long before diabetes was a part of our lives. Now it was personal.

At a campaign stop with my mother, Elle and I both got to meet actor Michael J. Fox, who had become a hero in the Parkinson's world and was one of the biggest national voices in favor of ending the stem-cell-research ban. Michael was one of my favorite actors. I'd grown up watching him on *Family Ties* and in movies like *Teen Wolf* and *Back to the Future*. It was exciting to meet him. But the celebrity side of it paled in comparison to the message he sent just by showing up.

Michael was having a rough day. His Parkinson's

medications weren't working as effectively as he would've liked, and it was difficult for him to stand and speak to that crowd full of television cameras and hundreds of students and spectators at the University of New Hampshire. Yet he'd flown all the way from Colorado—setting aside his own physical comfort and well-being in order to stand up for a cause that he believed in, a cause that he fully realized he may never see any direct benefit from in his own lifetime. For him, it was about fighting for the future. It was about fighting for other people. You could hear it in his words and see it on his face: Michael J. Fox found hope by focusing on the future and the promise of medical research. It seemed to me as if he found some relief from the burden of his illness by doing what he could to help shape the future for my daughter and millions of others who suffer every day with a chronic condition or debilitating disease.

After the event, Elle and I walked to Young's Restaurant, the family diner where my dad used to take me on Friday mornings before school to treat me to a chocolate milk and a cinnamon log while we practiced for my spelling tests. Elle sang show tunes all the way down Main Street, living out loud as she always did, but as we processed our big afternoon over lunch, Elle's questions turned to Parkinson's disease. "How close are they to finding a cure? What's Michael's prognosis? Will he ever get better?" she asked. Elle did the math, and through her questions I watched her come to understand that we'd had the privilege to witness a truly selfless act that day. "At least with diabetes," she declared, "we will find a cure in my lifetime."

This was the Shaheen gene in her, and just like my dad (the most optimistic man in America), Elle had the intuitive sense that you had to say it out loud in order to make it happen. Meeting Michael J. Fox and hearing him speak that day reinforced for her that having faith and using your voice are enormously important assets. And Elle knew that she had both. She had faith that things were going to get better in her lifetime, and she knew that her voice could help make a difference.

I was so proud of my daughter for wanting to be a force for change and a force for good herself. In a very short time following her diagnosis she saw her efforts, combined with the work of countless others over many years, lead to a significant victory: In early 2009, Elle and I were invited guests at the White House on the day President Barack Obama signed an executive order overturning the eight-year ban on human embryonic stem-cell research.

Elle was the only child in the room for that ceremony. She wore a light pink dress with her hair tied back, and I beamed with pride as I stood behind her and watched her shake hands with the president of the United States. It was breathtaking. My daughter was given the extraordinary gift of knowing that something good had come from her struggle and hard work. She was hooked.

From there the advocacy work we did together continued to build. One event would lead to another, then another meeting, another step forward.

Elle and I were both deeply involved with JDRF by then, and that spring, Elle was selected along with more than a hundred other kids from around the country to be a delegate to the JDRF's Children's Congress. The biannual event is widely considered the preeminent patient advocacy event in Washington. It's a spectacular program in which children living with diabetes share intimate exchanges with legislators, explaining to them what it's like to actually live with diabetes. These children break through all of the statistics and personalize diabetes for our country's senators and congressional leaders, one-on-one and as a powerful group.

Elle was thrilled when she got the invitation. "D.C., baby! Bring it!" she shouted in one of the many character voices her proud theater-geek mind created. "Elle's coming and she's got something to say, and y'all better listen!"

So that June, the two of us once again said good-bye to our family and headed down to Washington, D.C. Elle created a hand-drawn scrapbook of her life with diabetes, filled with pictures and memories of her diagnosis and the struggles she'd been through. She was able to show that scrapbook and talk about her experience with all four representatives from the state of New Hampshire, in their offices, one-on-one. She sat on the floor of a congressional hearing room, listening to a panel discuss legislation that would have a direct impact on her life and the lives of so many of her newfound peers. She even got to go to the White House again, where she met one of her idols, Nick Jonas—from platinum-selling music group the Jonas Brothers—who has type 1 himself. Meeting a young person who was a hugely successful performer not unlike she aspired to be one day had a huge impact on Elle's outlook about what was possible for her future. If it wasn't clear already, it became crystal clear to her during that trip that as long as we were vigilant, diabetes wouldn't hold her back. From anything.

Our attendance at that first Children's Congress opened the door to what we quickly learned was a gigantic network of families working feverishly to fight the devastating effects of diabetes. It wasn't just in conference rooms, either. We had meals together and took our kids to the pool back at the hotel. I remember Elle coming out of the pool at one point to check her blood sugar, and she was low—but this time every parent in the place could offer up a juice box or some kind of sugar to help! It was such a powerful, warm feeling to be in a place where everyone around us just *got it*. We met so many extraordinary people there who had dedicated their lives to curing this disease and who were doing everything they could to make life with diabetes more livable in the meantime.

Remembering their dedication and passion would give us hope and renew our spirits when times were especially difficult.

Through it all, I dug into the diabetes awareness world, attacking my research with the same vigor I'd applied at Harvard. What I didn't know astounded me. The consequences of diabetes extend well beyond the impact it has on those living with the disease. Diabetes takes a major toll on the U.S. economy. Directly and indirectly, the United States spent $174 billion on diabetes in 2007, a figure that is expected to triple in the next twenty-five years. One of every ten dollars spent on health care in this country goes to treat diabetes and its complications.

I also learned that whenever those statistics are reported, they combine type 1 and type 2, which causes a lot of confusion. It also astounded me just how little understanding the general public has of the difference between type 1 and type 2. Even extended family members would ask misguided questions like, "Is her diabetes under control?" or "Is it possible she'll grow out of it?"

Sometimes I wished type 1 had a completely different name, just to make it clear to people that it's an autoimmune disease—one that never goes away. A lot of people assume that a kid with diabetes has a parent

who let them eat all sorts of junk, as if that's what led
to the diagnosis. The misinformation made me want to
work even harder to raise awareness.

With each passing day, I watched my daughter blos-
som in her ever-growing shoes as a fighter for the most
personal cause imaginable. She began talking about
her diabetes more openly with friends. When asked
to speak in front of a class at school or elsewhere, she
jumped at the chance, and she treated those opportunities with the same sort of attention and enthusiasm
she would lend to her musical-theater performances
onstage.

Even though it was uncomfortable for her and
required another hospital stay, and even though it was
not clear whether she would feel a direct benefit from
the drug therapy, Elle was enthusiastic when the time
came for a second phase of her medical trial at Yale-
New Haven Hospital. After two more weeks out of
school, being poked and prodded, hooked up to monitors, and plagued by more blood tests than I could
imagine, she came home bursting with a greater desire
to volunteer for other clinical trials. She even managed to inspire every member of our family to donate
blood to researchers who are working on pinpointing
the genetic, hereditary components of diabetes.

Even with Elle's personal sacrifices and our joint
advocacy work on a national level, it didn't feel like
enough. The regulatory process was too slow to change.

Over the next couple of years, we'd find out that FDA regulations were primarily responsible for stopping investments in devices that could be life-changing— including an artificial pancreas—because inventors and investors could not identify a clear pathway to FDA approval. We learned that by 2010, medical devices were regularly being approved in Europe four full *years* ahead of devices in the United States—and the safety records of those devices remained comparable to devices in the United States, despite all the waiting. So U.S. companies had begun taking their business overseas, and patients from the United States were increasingly forced to travel overseas to find the cutting-edge care they wanted, needed, and deserved.

Facing that frustration while battling the same daily struggles, the inexplicable highs and lows, and the fight to adjust Elle's insulin doses not only for each meal, but also for every tiny change in her growing body, was difficult.

My heart grew heavy every time I tiptoed into Elle's room to quietly prick her finger with a lancet. The reality is that none of the promising research or medical advancements were ready yet. We tried everything we could get our hands on. Elle participated in other studies. We invested in the latest technology, from meters to test strips, and nothing made our day-to-day life much easier. There was not a single piece of technology or any sort of medical intervention that could provide our family immediate relief from the day-to-day stress and sometimes debilitating fear that Elle's blood sugar might drop so low that she'd have another seizure, or that it would spike so high that she'd wind up in a coma, or that the frequency of her high blood sugars might cause her to suffer the devastating long-term effects of this disease.

So we just kept searching.

The momentum of all of our endeavors reached a new peak when Elle and I were asked to co-chair the 2011 Children's Congress. The primary focus of that year's event would be regulatory reform, and suddenly all of our firsthand experience talking to concerned doctors and frustrated scientists felt like the perfect preparation. We enthusiastically accepted the invitation.

Oddly enough, as we began preparing for the event, we were forced to pay attention to a development outside of the worlds of science and medicine for the first time.

As co-chair, I was one of several committee members tasked with selecting that year's delegates, and of the hundreds of applications sent in by families with children who wanted to attend, a handful included long, passionate letters about their *dogs*. "Medic-alert dogs," they called them. "Diabetes dogs."

The letters spoke about the "life-changing effects" these dogs were having on their families. They opined on the talents of German shepherds, Labs, and golden retrievers that were apparently capable of sensing whenever their owner's blood sugar was getting too high or too low. They insisted that the dogs were capable of alerting the person living with diabetes or a parent whenever it happened.

They made it seem as if these dogs were miracle workers, but the skeptic in me wondered.

I remembered briefly hearing something about service dogs at the last Children's Congress, two years earlier. The concept seemed too far-fetched to take seriously, so I'd dismissed it out of hand. Now these families were applying and asking that their dogs be allowed to accompany them into the halls of Congress and the White House. The dogs, they insisted, were certified service animals covered by the Americans with Disabilities Act (ADA) guidelines, which technically meant that we couldn't refuse them access to the buildings or to any of JDRF's activities, just as organizations and businesses can't refuse seeing-eye dogs.

The ADA is robust, and of course no one at JDRF wanted to be accused of discriminating against any family dealing with diabetes. But would dogs be a distraction? How many delegates would want to bring a dog? Would we have issues with our transportation provider? Could we really bring dogs into the U.S. Capitol?

It was no small feat to have an animal qualified under the ADA. There had to be verifiable evidence that the dog was delivering a service that the person could not otherwise perform independently. The fact that the dogs were covered by ADA guidelines meant that they must be doing what these families said they were doing. I just couldn't believe it. It sounded far-fetched, and usually when something seems too good to be true, it is. Maybe the dogs provided companionship, and maybe they were well trained enough to help remind kids with diabetes to test themselves on a more regular basis. Or something. I had heard that dogs have a calming effect on human blood pressure. Maybe that was also a contributing factor to the positive effect these dogs seemingly had on kids with diabetes. Any of those things were a good and worthwhile reason for kids with diabetes to have a well-trained dog in their lives, but I couldn't imagine those dogs were truly capable of anything more.

What I chose to believe or not believe didn't really matter. There was no denying that medic-alert dogs were becoming a point of hope for a small segment of people living with diabetes. In the end, one young girl with a diabetes-alert dog was selected to be a delegate. I was nervous about how her dog would behave, of course, and the broader issue of whether an animal in our midst might distract from JDRF's core mission of increasing funding for diabetes research. I also wondered, *If this dog really can detect blood sugar levels and alert highs and lows, won't he go berserk and start*

barking and howling nonstop in a room full of hun-
dreds of people with diabetes?

I mentioned the letters we received from applicants with diabetes-alert dogs to Elle, but she didn't seem very interested. When I asked her if these dogs were something she wanted to look into, she shrugged her shoulders. Elle wasn't a big fan of dogs. She'd been bitten as a child, and even though Craig and I both love dogs, and her siblings—especially Annah—had been begging us to get a dog for ages, she just wasn't interested. That made it easy to put it out of my mind— until June came around, and something happened that opened my eyes.

Attending our second Children's Congress was as exciting and invigorating as it was the first time around. Maybe even more so. Reconnecting with so many families who struggled with day-to-day care just as we did was helpful, too. Craig was able to fly down and attend the event with us that time, while my sister took care of Annah, Caraline, and William. Elle was happy that her dad would not miss out on the experience this time, but having us both away from home also bothered her.

"I know this isn't fair," Elle said in the car on the way to the airport.

"What isn't fair?" Craig asked her.

"That both of you left just to come with me," she said.

"Elle, someday your sisters and brother will understand. It's not fair that you have diabetes. Sometimes life isn't fair," I said. "Even though they miss us and it's a lot to ask of our family, they do love staying with their aunts and uncles and cousins, you know."

"I guess," Elle said.

There were times when just by listening to the sound of her voice, I knew that Elle was acutely aware of just how much diabetes had taken from her family.

Once we were in Washington, however, the camaraderie with other parents who share so many of the same struggles was a helpful reminder that Craig and I weren't alone with our constant fear and worry. None of the other parents seemed to have found a solution to the anxiety, either, despite everything science and medicine had to offer.

Periodically I would see that little girl with her diabetes-alert dog, standing beside her mother going in or out of one of the workshops. It just felt so foreign to me. The very idea of diabetes-alert dogs made me wonder if perhaps some parents were buying into false hopes, simply because the pressure and anxiety of it all was so enormous. To me, putting hope and responsibility in the paws of a dog amounted to nothing more than clinging to that same false sense of security I'd managed to build in myself during Elle's first year after diagnosis. We all need something or someone to lean on. I just couldn't believe that an animal could do what science and technology could not.

There were more pressing things to focus on during our Washington trip, anyway, including a visit from Supreme Court Justice Sonia Sotomayor.

Supreme Court justices rarely make public appearances and aren't allowed to do anything political, so having her speak to the families gathered at the Children's Congress felt historic. Months earlier, Elle and I had learned that Justice Sotomayor was type 1, so we sat down together and wrote her a letter, asking her to speak. We were thrilled when she said yes.

My mother, Senator Jeanne Shaheen—who ran again and won in 2008—had a chance to meet and work with Justice Sotomayor during her confirmation, so it only made sense that she would join us to introduce Justice Sotomayor to the crowd. It also made sense that Elle, the one who had brought us here in the first place, would introduce her grandmother.

Justice Sotomayor's visit took place in a large conference room at the hotel we were all staying in, far from the eyes of the media that were covering many of the other Children's Congress events. The 100 child delegates all sat on the floor, with their parents crowded around the perimeter of the room. There were close to 300 people in the room when Elle took to the podium. She stood tall and proud and talked about how grateful she was to her grandmother for being so supportive and helping to fight for diabetes research.

"One day we will all benefit from that," Elle said, "because one day there will be a cure. And between now and then, things will happen that will make our lives better."

She also noted how honored she was to have Justice Sotomayor there because they shared something bitter-sweet: They were both diagnosed with type 1 at the age of eight.

Justice Sotomayor didn't stand at the podium that day. She sat in an armchair so she could talk to the children in a comfortable, less-intimidating position. She spoke eloquently about her own struggle with diabetes, but it wasn't until one particular little girl asked a question from the audience that the tears started to flow. This little five-year-old from South Carolina stood up and asked, in the sweetest Southern accent, "Miss Justice, can you tell me if it ever gets any easier?"

Justice Sotomayor took a moment. Then she opened up about the most personal aspects of her struggle. She reminded the audience that she was diagnosed at age eight, like Elle, and that her parents worked, which meant that she had to administer her own insulin. They didn't have disposable syringes in those days. Instead she had a special stool that she would climb up on in order to place her reusable needles in a pot to be boiled and sanitized. Those needles were big, she said, and thick. There were no spring-loaded lancets with which to prick her finger, either. She had to use a razor blade to do the job. Kids all over that room gasped at the very thought of it.

"But medical advances do happen," she said, "and things do get better over time."

There was that phrase again. That notion: *Things do get better.*

I quietly prayed more fervently than ever that those words were true.

Finally, at the Childen's Congress closing event, Craig and I again took note of that little girl with her sweet dog, sitting in the well of the U.S. Senate committee hearing room. The children were gathered front and center, seated on the floor of a dark wood-paneled room, while parents took a backseat in the galleys along the perimeter. That dog sat ever so patiently at the girl's feet, even in the middle of a large crowd, surrounded by dozens of cameras while a series of JDRF representatives, including some of the kids, shared testimony with members of the Senate. I could hardly believe how well behaved this dog was, given the circumstances. Despite all of the activity happening around him, he sat quietly and attentively. I never knew a dog that could walk into a room full of people without running around and sniffing everyone or barking at something for seemingly no reason or jumping up to say hi. Not this dog. This dog impressed me.

Elle was sitting close to the girl and her dog, and I saw her look over when suddenly the dog sat straight up. He scanned the crowded room looking for the girl's mother. When he couldn't find her, he started circling around the child to get her mother's attention. Soon the mom was at her daughter's side. She whispered something to her. The girl pulled out her lancet and test kit and checked right there in the middle of the hearing room. Her dog kept pacing. Sure enough, her blood sugar was out of range! I wasn't close enough to discern if she was high or low, but they made their adjustments, rewarded the dog, and he lay right back down. The incident was over in a matter of seconds. They didn't even disturb the hearing. It was stunning.

This little girl would never have tested in the middle of a hearing room if the dog hadn't grabbed her mother's attention. The room was quiet. It was a serious place. Even if she weren't feeling good, chances are she would've waited to test until the hearing was over and she was back with her parents. What if her blood sugar was dropping fast? A half-hour difference could mean a seizure. That dog's action caused her to test, and therefore treat, long before it would have happened otherwise.

I made a mental note to myself: *I need to learn more about these dogs!*

CHAPTER 7

A Distant Howl

"How do dogs help people see? Well, if you are blind, you don't need just a person to help. You can have a dog help you."

—"What Dogs Do for People," by Elle, age 7

As soon as I got back home to New Hampshire, I started looking into the growing field of medic-alert dogs. The whole concept was relatively new, so there was no one national organization to turn to for information. There didn't appear to be any regulations. There were no standard protocols. It was a frustrating search for answers because things were disaggregated. Still, from what I could gather, the training protocols for these animals were adapted from the training methods used for narcotics-detection, search-and-rescue, and cadaver-detection dogs. One training protocol in particular was developed by an individual with diabetes who happened to be a certified trainer of dogs for search-and-rescue and narcotics detection. Understanding the cues and scents dogs pick up on, he decided to see if the dogs could sense changes in blood sugar or body chemistry in order to prevent his own life-threatening situations. Lo and behold, he found that the dogs could do exactly what he desired, and more.

Slowly, word spread. People started nonprofit and for-profit businesses exploiting and maximizing the potential that dogs seem to have to help humans in previously unheard of ways. Before long, there were dogs out there helping to prevent epileptic seizures, alerting people to heart attacks and spikes in blood pressure, helping combat veterans deal with PTSD, and even sniffing out various types of cancer.

It all seemed to gather steam in a grassroots way, and without much scientific study. The evidence that dogs could actually accomplish these things seemed entirely anecdotal. Still, it was pretty overwhelming. The more I searched, the more I found story after story of dogs saving lives.

The ability for dogs to sense these specific changes in humans seemed to come down to the canine's extraordinary sense of smell. An average dog's sensitivity to smell is 10,000 to 100,000 times more powerful than a human's. It's difficult for us to even comprehend what this means, but while humans pick up scent in parts per million, dogs can smell odors in parts per *trillion*. The PBS show *NOVA* did a special about this in which they drew an analogy to human sight: If a dog's ability to see were 10,000 times more powerful than ours, then whatever we could see at 1/3 of a mile, a dog could see just as clearly from more than 3,000 miles away. *Three thousand miles!* The show also contended that while we humans might be able to detect a teaspoon of sugar in a cup of coffee, a dog could detect a teaspoon of sugar in a *million gallons* of coffee.

When it comes to sniffing out changes in blood sugar for people living with diabetes, trainers use saliva taken from diabetics at various blood-glucose readings. The saliva samples, on cotton swabs, are frozen to store and thawed for use during the training process. Over time, dogs are trained to recognize the smell of blood glucose in the normal 80 to 120 range and to differentiate that scent from the dangerous lows and highs.

The more I read, the more it made sense to me how this might actually work.

Still, I was skeptical. Everyone's body chemistry is different, and it still didn't make sense to me that a dog could tackle a job that medical science hadn't yet mastered. I'd seen the results with my own eyes, though, and Craig and I decided it was time to talk about it as a family.

Of course, mentioning the word *dog* in my household led to much pleading, with Annah, our animal lover, leading the charge. "When are we getting a dog?" she kept asking from the moment I brought it up.

Part of me wanted to get a dog just to make Annah happy, almost as much as I wanted to get a dog with the potential to help Elle. Even if a medic-alert dog didn't turn out to be a wonder dog capable of fighting diabetes, I figured at the very least he or she might be a well-trained dog, and *that* might help me to forget about a terrible, no-good, very bad mistake I'd made not so long ago.

After Elle had her seizure on her one-year diaversary, I was terrified. Frankly, I was a mess. I felt completely overwhelmed. Everything seemed hard, all the time, and I just needed something *good* to happen. I received an e-mail from a friend one day containing an adorable picture of a brand-new litter of yellow Lab puppies, and I declared, "That's it. We're getting the kids a new puppy for Christmas."

Craig and I had a yellow Lab before we had kids. That dog was like our first baby. I'd grown up with dogs. My parents raised Old English sheepdogs and I'd gotten a dog of my own when I was eleven. Our kids *should* have a dog, and I was absolutely convinced that a new puppy would bring some magic back into our family.

The puppy arrived in a box with a bow on Christmas morning, and the kids were thrilled. They named him Ebenezer. That's right. As in "Scrooge."

Well, Eben, as we called him, turned out to be a

disaster. In the course of just a few months, he grew to 120 pounds. He kept knocking our newly toddling William right over. He yanked so hard on the leash that the kids couldn't take him for walks. Actually, Craig could barely take him for walks. We didn't have the time or space to train him the way he needed to be trained or to give him the effort any rambunctious Lab deserves, so he tore up pillows and shoes and his fair share of beloved stuffed animals. Elle, especially, wanted nothing to do with him. She was constantly annoyed by his unpredictability, his jumping, his nipping. Even animal-loving Annah grew tired of his antics.

In the end, all that dog did was make our lives more stressful. So we gave him up. It broke my heart, but we found a family friend, a landscaper who loves that dog to pieces and who gave him a wonderful home. He brings Eben with him in his pickup to job sites, and they're together and outdoors all day long. Eben's as happy as a yellow Lab could be now. I'm still embarrassed and sorry that we weren't able to make it work.

The weight of my terrible, impulsive decision in our recent past certainly weighed heavily on any new thoughts I had about getting a dog, even a medic-alert dog with the potential to help our daughter.

Then I saw the cost. One organization charged $25,000—for a *dog*. There was absolutely no way we could afford that, even if there was rock-solid proof that these dogs were miracle workers.

Just as the hope of that miracle seemed to mostly slip away, I came across a newspaper article from Georgia highlighting the experience of one young boy living with diabetes. I recognized his name. He had applied to be a delegate to the Children's Congress. The piece referenced an organization in Kansas called CARES— a nonprofit that trains medic-alert dogs for diabetes and seizure alert, along with PTSD and a number of other conditions.

I decided to give the idea one more shot, and I called CARES. The first question I asked was how much it cost, and I found out directly from the organization's founder, a delightful woman named Sarah, that the cost of one of their dogs was around $2,500, fully trained. That was ten times more feasible a price for us, and my interest piqued all over again.

Sarah explained that their dogs were trained with a multistep process to ensure a high success rate. CARES begins their work with new litters of puppies—all of whom are donated by their various breeders—and hand-selects the dogs best suited to medic-alert work. Those puppies are then placed with volunteer families for the first few months of life, where they are socialized and housebroken and where some initial training begins. The dogs then move from the care of the families to the care of specially trained inmates at a nearby prison rehabilitation program. The inmates, who are all nonviolent offenders, go through extensive training and have to meet certain criteria. They are then put in charge of teaching commands while also acclimating the dogs to handle a regimented schedule and long days. A medic-alert dog will often have to sit or stay for hours at a time, Sarah explained, and what better environment than a prison to instill that sort of discipline?

The very nature of an inmate-trainer–dog relationship means that the dogs help the prisoners while the prisoners train the dogs. I admired that. I also admired that the training was provided at no additional cost to CARES. That helped keep CARES' overhead low, and that savings was passed on to families like mine. A win-win scenario all around.

The final stage in the approximately eighteen-month-long cycle brought the dogs to CARES for specialized training in the particular field they'd be working in. Then it was their mission to get those dogs into the hands of those who needed their services.

Hearing all of that made it actually feel like a possibility to me.

I didn't want to repeat past mistakes, so I didn't rush. I called CARES multiple times to inquire about what it would be like to bring one of their dogs into our big family. The thing they assured me was that, in addition to doing the job they'd been trained for, any of their dogs would be extremely well mannered. We wouldn't be getting a pillow-shredding untrained puppy all over again.

Because CARES invests so much in these animals, they also told me they want to ensure that each placement is a success. So within six months, if you get home and the relationship isn't working, CARES reserves the right to reclaim the dog. On the flip side, we would have the ability in the first six months to give the dog back if we didn't think it was working out for us. The dog would then be placed with another family. They also said they would refund a percentage of our money if that happened, since they could place the dog with another family.

There seemed to be very little downside.

"Worst-case scenario," I told Craig, "is we're out some money and some time."

We decided it was time for a family meeting.

Elle was aggravated that we didn't talk to her first before talking about it in front of her siblings.

"Yes, yes, yes, we want a dog!" they all yelled the moment the words came from my lips. I recognized later that this did put unfair pressure on Elle to say yes. But the more we talked about it together, the more she came around.

"Guys, if you think this will help, I'll try it," she said. "Just remember that my track record with dogs isn't very good. I mean, I'll go along with it, but—"

"Yay!" Annah and Caraline and William all squealed.

I was still hesitant. I wasn't sure we were ready. I

still wasn't over the sting of giving up on Eben. If we were going to do this, we would have to work hard to make sure the dog would become a part of our family. We *had* to make this work.

Then came the clincher: I called CARES back and was told they had a waiting list of eighteen to twenty-four months for each dog. That seemed plenty long enough to hold the kids off for a while and yet satisfy them with the idea that a dog would be coming eventually. It would also give us some time to let the kids get a little bit older, so they'd be better equipped to help care for a dog in our home. *And* it would give me enough time to hopefully get used to the idea of having one more mouth to feed in our chaotic household.

CARES only required a hundred-dollar deposit to hold a spot. I was still skeptical, and so was Elle. But the idea that a dog might actually encourage her to check her blood sugar more frequently seemed like a bonus given that we'd also be getting a well-trained dog with the potential to become a beloved member of our family.

It didn't feel like a big commitment to me. It felt like a *gradual* commitment. And that was a commitment I was willing to make.

CHAPTER 8

Lessons Learned

"Maybe it would be like a vacation. Maybe my mom could sleep through the night. I have so much responsibility on me now. I don't know any other 12-year-old close to me who has that big a responsibility on them. I want a carefree childhood."

—Elle, age 12

Thoughts of a new dog joining our family all but disappeared as we turned the corner into 2012. The deposit was made and the kids were excited, but we knew it wouldn't happen for quite some time.

It was difficult for me to believe that Elle, my first baby, was twelve years old, and even harder for me to believe that she'd be a teenager come September. There were times when I'd catch a glimpse of her from a certain angle and be completely shocked by how grown up she looked. She was tall, almost as tall as me now—a fact that she made a point to remind me of, regularly. She was in middle school. She was acting in the professional setting of the Seacoast Repertory Theatre on an almost continuous basis now, tackling everything from *The Diary of Anne Frank* to her favorite song-and-dance numbers in Broadway-style musical-theater shows, including *Annie, Guys and Dolls*, and *The Sound of Music*. There was even the occasional mention of boys when she and her friends hung out together after school, in that telling tone that signaled the impending, inevitable coming of adolescence.

The milestones in her ability to care for her diabetes kept coming, too. She was not only self-testing now, but after years of practice I finally grew comfortable letting her self-dose insulin, as long as she made sure to ask for help figuring out how much to take if she had questions about the nutrients in a given meal or snack. She could rattle off the number of carbs in the standard snacks, including apples, carrots, and yogurt, as quickly as I could.

I still had to help her insert the pump site and would occasionally have to make a trip to the school if the site fell out during the day. But for the most part, my physical duty of testing and treating Elle was relegated to the overnight shift.

The freedom allowed me to dedicate some time to a new idea: cofounding a company that could make things

easier for anyone living with a nutrition-sensitive medical condition. The concept was to bring technology and
service together in a way that would help make it easier
for individuals and families to figure out their specific
dietary needs given food preferences, chronic conditions, and lifestyle preferences. The journey would be
a long one, but eventually my business partner George
Bennett and I launched Good Measures, LLC. Soon I
was commuting to Boston twice a week to try to get
this company off the ground.

Of course, as any parent of a child with type 1 will
attest, I was always checking the clock and wondering
when Elle last tested or took insulin, and I constantly
worried about her blood sugar. We had multiple conversations each day about how much insulin she'd taken.
I still had a better handle on how much insulin she
should take, given the foods she planned to eat. There
were times when she'd call me from school, and I'd
serve as her guide: "I think you should treat for thirty
grams of carb, set a temporary basal for three hours at
120 percent. And you need to recheck in two hours."
Then I would explain the same thing to the adult in
charge at the time.

The fact that a twelve-year-old and her various
caregivers understood what any of that complicated
language meant shows just how far we'd all come. Yet I
was still the mother with my list of questions each and
every time she walked out of the house, each and every

time she left for rehearsal, each and every time she left for dance class, and each and every time she finished whatever activity she'd been doing. Before school. After school...

"*Mom!*" she'd complain in that exasperated tone that tweens seem to master so effortlessly. Still, I would not stop. I'd heard horror stories about tweens and teens skipping their checking because they didn't want to feel embarrassed in front of their peers or deal with the hassle. Kids generally don't want to be different. They just want to fit in and be "normal," and we'd already experienced that in the worst way the first time Elle went off to a sleepover summer camp.

I'll never forget the panic I felt when the camp's nurse, who also happened to be our neighbor, called from all those many miles away to let me know that Elle was vomiting, suffering from a horrible headache, and her color was off. We'd put protocols in place to make sure the camp counselors and the adults who worked with her checked in with Elle about her blood glucose readings multiple times each day and night. But it turned out that Elle was making up numbers. She wasn't actually checking. She didn't want to appear different from the other kids and didn't want to slow down enough to stop what she was doing and test. She didn't think it would be that big of a deal. *How bad could things get in a couple of days?* she thought. As a result, within two days her blood sugars were through the roof. She wound up suffering the effects of ketoacidosis.

Elle was ten when that happened. I'd agonized over whether to let her go. I'd spent countless hours working with nurses and camp counselors before she went and while she was there. I probably wouldn't have let her go if our neighbor, who also served as the school nurse at our local high school, wasn't going to be there. Elle wanted to go to camp to prove that she could handle it, in the hopes that we'd eventually let her go to a prestigious theater camp she'd heard about that was many states away. She almost blew her chance in the first two days, but we both learned a hard lesson—a lesson that stuck. She'd gone to camp each summer since, including to that prestigious summer theater camp of her dreams, with no further incidents. She proved that she could responsibly manage the daily regimen required of diabetes.

Now that she was almost a teen, I prayed that her earlier behavior would not be repeated.

Elle had done fairly well during her first four years AD. Her A1C tests were never quite as low as we wanted them to be, but certainly not as high as some of the horror stories we'd heard. On average she still had more highs and lows from day to day than anyone would like, and Dr. Ricker reminded us that an elevated A1C could lead to long-term complications (not

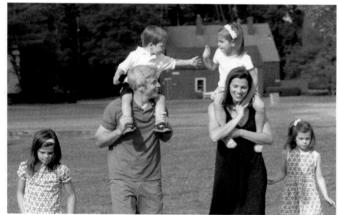

Four kids under age eight made life before diabetes busy—but beautiful.

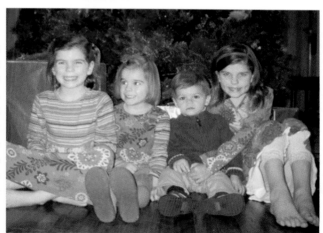

Elle (right) was diagnosed the day after this photo was taken at the Mount Washington Hotel. With Annah (far left), Caraline, and William.

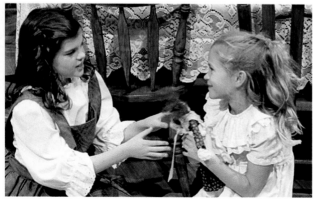

Following the diagnosis, Elle clung to her love of the performing arts, insisting, "The show must go on" even in the face of a major medical emergency. Here she is on stage just hours after being hospitalized following a major seizure.

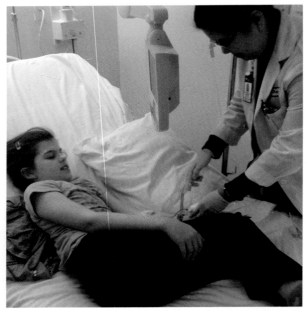

Elle wanted to be part of the search for a cure, so she decided to participate in clinical trials, including this one at Yale-New Haven Hospital.

Inspired by advocates for medical research, including Michael J. Fox, Elle and I actively added our voices to the cause. Craig snapped this shot of Elle proudly sharing her new insulin pump.

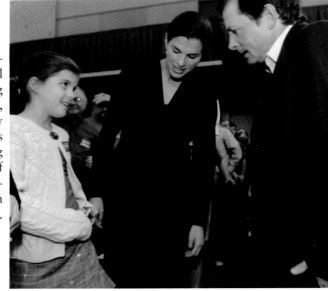

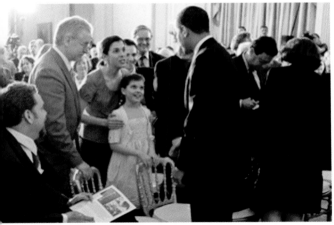

Our advocacy work led us to the White House for President Obama's signing of an executive order to restore critical medical research.

Elle joined a chorus of delegates at the Juvenile Diabetes Research Foundation Children's Congress, where she told members of Congress, including her grandmother, U.S. Senator Jeanne Shaheen, what it is like to live with diabetes.

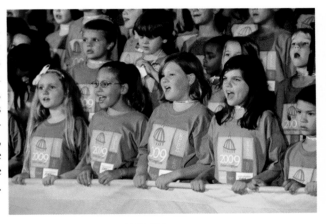

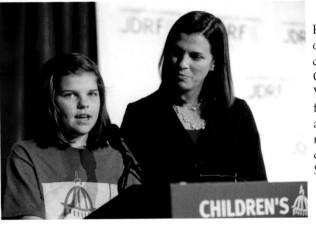

Elle and I had the opportunity to co-chair the 2011 Children's Congress. What a proud moment for us to take the stage and introduce my mom, who then welcomed Justice Sonia Sotomayor!

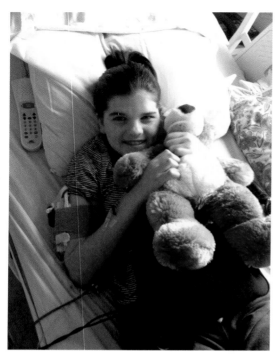

Elle was one of the first children to test an artificial pancreas device at Mass General Hospital. It was hard to say goodbye to this technology at the end of the clinical trial because it is still years away from coming home with us.

Elle meets Coach! This was right at the beginning of the training process, on one of their first public outings together in Kansas.

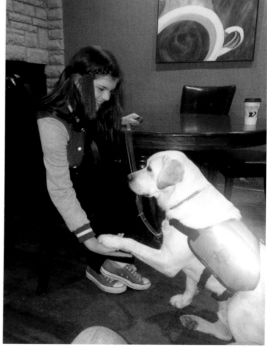

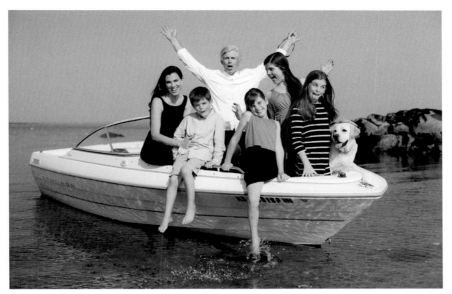

Bringing Coach home to join our family gave us all reason to celebrate!

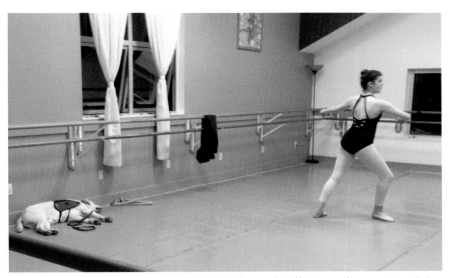

Coach quickly learned to paw his way through Elle's regular routine, joining her for dance class, voice lessons, and theater rehearsals.

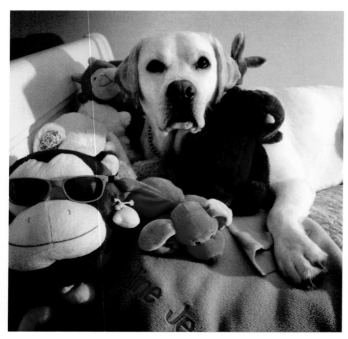

Coach became a
helpful part of the
bedtime routine in
our house.

Elle and Coach
are worn out
after a long day
of theater camp,
but it is reassur-
ing to always
have Coach along
for the ride.

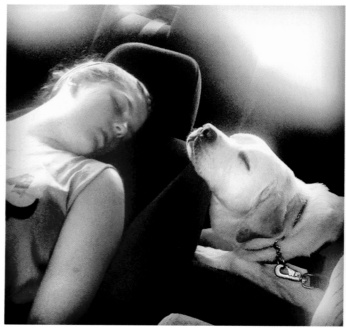

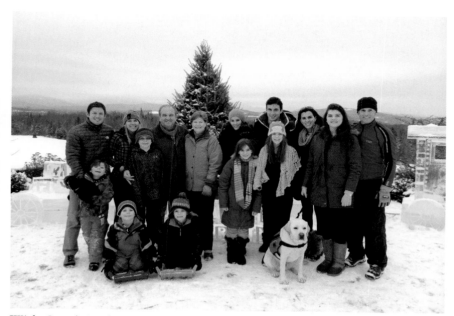

With Coach in the picture, this 2013 trip up north with my parents, my sisters, and their families felt like a world away from our visit the weekend before Elle's diagnosis.

Dropping my little girl and Coach off for their first day of high school was a bitter-sweet day. Where does the time go?

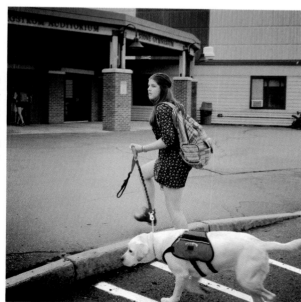

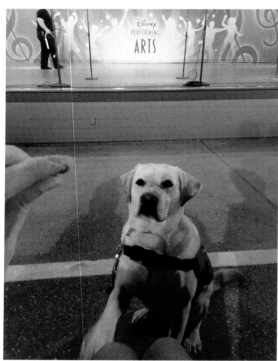

A few minutes before Elle was set to take this Disney stage for a performance with Boston Children's Theatre, Coach alerted me by pawing my lap because her blood sugar was too high. Good boy, Coach!

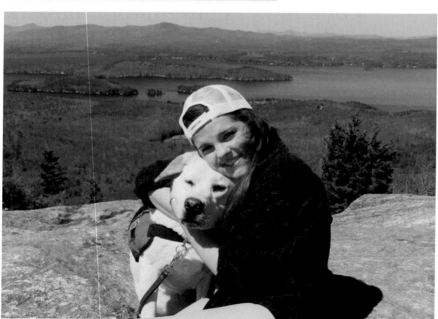

What a team! This dynamic duo is going places together.

to mention that the dramatic fluctuations made Elle feel awful). We still needed to do better, but she hadn't suffered a seizure since her first diaversary, and other than the one ketoacidosis incident at summer camp, she'd done well avoiding the extreme highs, too. That was something to celebrate.

We had something exciting to look forward to in the fall that year as well. Our insurance would finally allow Elle to upgrade her insulin pump, and we were in line to set her up with a pump that connected to a continuous glucose monitor. The technological advances we'd dreamed of were slowly becoming a reality, and we hoped that a continuous monitor would finally make managing her insulin doses less of a mathematical guessing game.

There was another advancement, too.

In the spring of 2012, Elle became the youngest-ever patient to participate in a clinical trial of an artificial pancreas—and it worked. For four whole days she didn't have to test her blood sugar. Elle didn't have to inject herself with insulin. Elle didn't have to think about what she ate, and neither did I. Unfortunately, she was confined to a hospital bed, connected to a twisting bundle of tubes and wires, unable to go about any of her normal daily activities. The device was several generations away from being portable. Still, for the first time since 2007, my daughter was able to take a four-day vacation from diabetes. The thought of it still brings tears to my eyes.

That trial was big enough news in the medical world that we got calls from CNN and the television show *The Doctors*, asking us to share Elle's story. Both of those national news and television outlets produced segments about Elle's experience, and our family, and what it meant to be a child living with type 1.

Elle's openness in front of the cameras was extraordinary. When CNN came to our home, they filmed her testing her blood sugar. When it came time to change her pump site, I offered to take her into the bathroom where the cameras couldn't follow, since a part of her lower back would be exposed in the process.

"Mom, if we're going to show people, we need to show them everything!" she insisted.

Not everything, I thought to myself. But this time we changed the pump site with the cameras rolling, using that big needle and inserting the site into the skin at her waist.

In the hospital, she pulled up her shirt to show the four continuous glucose monitors and the tangled web of wires and tubes attached to her stomach that they were testing as part of the artificial pancreas, too.

Then they brought Elle and me on for live interviews. I was nervous going on live TV, worried about what I'd say, worried that I'd cry on national television as I spoke about my daughter and the difference an artificial pancreas could make in Elle's life, and in mine. Elle didn't seem nervous at all. After leaving at 4:30 a.m. for the drive to CNN's satellite studio outside of Boston, she sat right down full of confidence and looked into the camera as if she'd done it a thousand times.

"Live TV is just like live theater," she told me. "We just need to get it right the first time."

She spoke eloquently about her condition in a way that earned praise from producers behind the scenes. These were professionals who dealt with people on both sides of the camera all day every day, and they all called Elle "a natural."

The appearance on *The Doctors* even afforded us a trip to L.A., where we were able to visit with my youngest sister. She took Elle to "finally" get her ears pierced—on the Sunset Strip in Hollywood, no less. For a preteen, it was like Disney and Christmas all rolled into one. I was amazed once more at the opportunities this unexpected journey gave to our family.

Having a taste of life without testing and carb counting and insulin was both a blessing and curse, though. Coming back home after that whirlwind made every finger prick and needle stick even more tiresome. Elle seemed more annoyed than ever by me and all of my questions.

Annah, Caraline, and William were affected by it, too. They all carried a fear that they might develop diabetes. They dreaded coming to Joslin with us for their annual blood tests. Especially William. I'm not sure if it's because of his physical resemblance to Elle or if it's just because he's the youngest and saw me testing his sisters, but he'd developed a penchant for asking me to check his blood sugar on a regular basis. I obliged, and so far he's always tested within the acceptable range, but still, knowing that he carries that worry is distressing. I hold my breath every time I prick his finger. And every time one of the kids seems especially thirsty or complains of a headache, the other kids make sure to tell me about it so I'll test them just in case.

One day Elle said to me, "I hate that they have a higher risk because of me."

"Elle," I said, "they don't have a higher risk *because* of you. The fact that you have diabetes just means we need to watch for it, because they're at risk, too. It's not *because* of you."

I hoped she hadn't been carrying that misunderstanding around since the beginning, and I hoped that my explanation provided some relief if she had.

New test strips, new medications, a new lancet recommended by Dr. Ricker or our CDE...it was amazing how anything "new" would give us a little lift. It was in many ways like buying new shoes. It would put a spring in our steps. But that feeling would never last. One of the biggest advances we were anticipating was the continuous glucose monitor (CGM). We all kept talking about how much we were looking forward to that device finally making things easier.

Then it didn't.

Wearing an early generation CGM in addition to the insulin pump made Elle feel like she was walking into a fashion show wearing a fanny pack. In her mind, she stuck out in all the wrong ways, which was the very last thing she wanted to do as an eighth grader. Life with the pump was awkward enough at times. She'd walk out of a theater performance with a bulge under her shirt and a stage manager would yell after her, "Hey, you forgot to take off your mic pack!"

"No," Elle would point out, "it's just my insulin pump."

Wearing two devices was that much more noticeable, cumbersome, and uncomfortable. The CGM meant a second site inserted with a large needle. Plus, it was difficult to calibrate and rarely accurate. When the CGM alerted her to a high or a low, she'd test the old-fashioned way and get a completely different reading, which made it more confusing than helpful most of the time. There was simply too much unreliable data for her to deal with. Elle wanted to do the right thing, to take the best care possible, but very quickly it seemed that the device was only making life harder.

The monitor also alerted her to every high and low with a beeping noise, like a pager. She kept beeping in the middle of math class, interrupting the teacher and making everyone turn their heads. It was embarrassing for Elle and distracting to everyone.

Lastly, it wasn't improving anything. At a regular checkup with Dr. Ricker, Elle wound up with one of her highest A1C results yet.

Dr. Ricker, in her direct way, said, "Elle, how can we help you?"

Elle cried when we left her office. She was angry that after all the aggravation of living with the CGM her blood work was getting worse, not better, and she was sick and tired of dealing with it. So six weeks in, she gave it up.

All those hopes and dreams of a little relief, something better, something easier, went away. Once again, life went right back to the way it was before.

CHAPTER 9

Flying Coach

"I am going to take a chance on this crazy idea for
my mom and for my family."

—Elle, age 13

The phone call caught me off guard.

"Hi there. It's Sarah, from CARES. I have some exciting news. Your dog is almost ready!"

It was the middle of January 2013, and the dog they'd picked out for us had just entered the final training phase. Elle and a parent would have to go to Kansas in March for a five-day in-person training session, where Elle would learn everything she needed to know to manage the dog, and if everything went according to plan, the pair would get certified as a licensed service team, Sarah explained. At the end of the five days, Elle and her dog would have to pass a public access test. They would go to a local mall and perform a series of tasks to demonstrate that they were comfortable working with each other, that the dog was attentive and responsive to Elle, and that Elle was able to manage the dog in a public setting.

"Are you excited?" she asked me.

"Yes," I said, hoping she didn't notice my hesitation.

"All right, then. We'll see Elle in March!"

Oh my God.

I had put it so far out of my mind I had almost forgotten that we might soon have a dog in the house. My mind flooded with images of carrying big bags of dog food home from the supermarket, worries about the financial cost and the time it took to schedule visits to the vet, not to mention the emergencies when a dog would inevitably get sick, and the walks he would need every day in the rain, sleet, snow, and wind just to go to the bathroom. We didn't have a yard in which we could just let him out to do his thing. Then there were the messes, the paw prints, the shedding, the wet dog smell when it rained.

Did the dog have a name? What kind of dog was it? We'd been told from the beginning that selecting a certain color, breed, and gender would further delay the process. We'd requested a Lab. We'd requested a male. But we said we'd be open to anything. Once the initial deposit was made, we didn't hear from CARES. The organization kept overhead low by limiting communication. They didn't send pictures of the dog as a puppy or provide any other info. It would all be a surprise.

I shared the news with Craig, and he seemed to take it in stride. "Oh, that's great!" he said. He'd just started a new job with the local public housing authority, so he was working close by now, and the idea that the dog might make the job of caring for Elle's diabetes a little easier on us seemed encouraging to him. I was surprised at how excited he seemed, given the disruption I was anticipating. He clearly saw the weight I carried and was far more optimistic than I was that a dog might actually help Elle out.

When we finally broke the news, the kids all squealed with delight. William was so young he barely remembered Eben at all, so to him, this was really going to feel like his first dog. Caraline was thrilled at the idea that she was potentially old enough now to walk a dog, and to groom it, and play fetch with it. And Annah was just beside herself. For her this was a dream come true.

Even Elle seemed excited if a little wary at the idea of going to Kansas and having to pass a test. She suddenly felt a lot of pressure, as if it was up to her to make sure that this dog actually made it home. The last thing she wanted was to let her siblings down. She didn't seem to be worried that the dog would bite her or anything. She seemed to trust the idea that this would be a "well-trained dog." But she questioned whether this dog would make any difference in her daily life. Nothing else had worked. Why would this?

She began to process her anxiety out loud by asking us all sorts of questions: "Will I be missing school?" "What if we don't pass the test?" "When do we have to leave?" "Who is going?"

Annah tried to jump in on that last one and happily volunteered to make the trip to Kansas. "After all, I love dogs more than anyone in the family," she said.

Unfortunately, we told her, no other kids were allowed.

We decided that Craig should be the parent who accompanied Elle to Kansas. He was able to manage it with his work schedule, and he also saw it as a good opportunity to spend time one-on-one with his oldest daughter. He didn't get that very often in our hectic, kid-juggling existence. Plus, I was still in start-up mode with Good Measures and had meetings in Boston that simply couldn't be canceled.

My nervousness that this whole thing might be a mistake only grew over the course of the next two months and seemed to be matched in our household by the growing excitement that kept overflowing from the three younger kids.

We weren't sure if the dog would have a name when we got it or if CARES would allow us to name the dog ourselves, which led to lots of discussion and debate. Craig wondered how we could live with a dog if we didn't like its name. How could he stand up and yell for that dog at a park if its name were Cupcake or Snuggles? A dog needed a good strong name, he insisted. We thought we ought to come up with a name we could all agree on, and the kids argued about it endlessly until we thought we'd finally settled on "Columbo." The kids liked imagining that service dog as a detective, and if it was a girl, they could shorten the name to just "Bo." Caraline then complained that it was outrageous to call a girl dog "Bo," and that discussion got William riled up about how important it was that the dog be a boy, because boys were already outnumbered in our family. So around and around the arguments went.

Then, a few days before Craig and Elle were set to fly out, everything went into slow motion.

Craig's father died.

While he had not been in good health, his death was still unexpected. Suddenly every plan we'd made took a backseat to grief and tears. Planning for a dog's arrival was quickly eclipsed by preparing ourselves for a funeral.

I called CARES to let them know what had happened and to ask about our options. Unfortunately, our options were limited. The training cycle for the dogs is intense and precise. If we couldn't pick up our dog this time around, they would give the dog to another family and we'd have to go back on the wait list. It could be another year before they'd have a dog available. Craig and I agreed that we simply could not let that happen. We couldn't do that to the kids. He and Elle were supposed to arrive in Kansas that Sunday to meet the dog and begin training. The wake was now scheduled for that day, and the funeral and burial on Monday. We checked into flights and asked if it was possible for Craig and Elle to fly in on Tuesday instead.

CARES had never made an exception to their protocol before. They were reluctant to do it. "Every hour of that training week is crucial," Sarah told me. There was a big long pause and I thought it was over. I thought we would be forced to wait another year.

"But you know," she said, "this dog we have picked out for you is really something special. He's just something else. He's already been on two planes and he handled it fine, and he finished his initial training ahead of schedule. We can give it a try."

"Oh, thank you. Thank you. This will mean so much to my family," I said.

"Just fair warning, if they aren't able to pass the public access test on Friday, that dog can't come home with you. We *can't* bend that rule," Sarah said.

"I understand. We'll do our best. Thank you. They'll see you on Tuesday for sure, and they will come ready to work," I said.

∽✖✎

I set my alarm for three o'clock that morning to make sure Craig and Elle got off to the airport okay. We had learned by then that stress was a factor that could wreak havoc on Elle's health, and this day was going to be plenty stressful. A surprise March snowstorm rolled in the night before, and from the look of it, the roads were going to be a mess. I checked and saw that the flight wasn't canceled. It wasn't even delayed. So I woke them both up and did all of the last-minute packing list checks before hugs and kisses and then they were off.

They encountered multiple accidents en route to Logan Airport, complete with emergency vehicles redirecting traffic onto side roads. After arriving late and barely making their flight, they wound up sitting on the runway for two hours with delays for deicing.

They were late enough that they were going to miss their connection, so I hopped on the phone and switched their next flight for them before getting our little ones off for their days and heading to Boston for a day full of meetings. I tried to keep in contact with Craig as much as I could, but I felt a bit like the ground crew for Apollo 13, waiting through hours and hours of nervous silence between updates.

When they finally arrived in Wichita, that tiny airport was out of rental cars.

"But I have a reservation," Craig said.

"You did have a reservation, but you didn't show up. We gave the car away, and we're out of cars now," the associate responded.

At that point, Craig channeled *me*: "I've been up since three a.m., stuck on runways, switching flights, all trying to get my daughter the help she needs, and I am not going to be stopped by a rental car company that claims it doesn't have any cars, when that's the only business you're in!"

Like magic, a car suddenly appeared. Someone apparently had "just returned it," the associate told him. It hadn't been washed yet. But Craig and Elle hopped into that dirty car and began the three-hour drive to their ultimate destination in north-central Kansas.

"There's nothing here, Dad," Elle said as they drove. "It's barren."

"I've never seen anything like it," Craig remarked of the seemingly endless flat terrain.

It was four in the afternoon when they finally stepped foot into a large room in a small-town church basement in Concordia where the CARES training classes were taking place. They'd missed most of another full day because of the snow and delays.

The class was in full swing when Craig and Elle poked their heads in. They were surprised to see fifteen dogs in that room, all paired up with people of various ages. There were Labs and golden retrievers and German shepherds, and every one of those dogs sat patiently and quietly at their handler's side. It was quite a sight.

They didn't want to interrupt, so they just listened. Oddly enough, that portion of the instruction was focused on grieving—talking to the dog recipients about the notion that someday these companion dogs would pass away and that the dogs' owners would need to be prepared for that.

Craig whispered to Elle, "Do we really have to learn how to grieve for it when we haven't even *met* the dog yet?"

Elle laughed at that. The entire trip had been exhausting and surreal for both of them.

Finally one of the instructors noticed them in the doorway and asked them to step out into the hall. "Oh, I'm so glad you finally made it. Stay put, now. We have your dog right here!" she said.

Elle looked up at her dad all wide-eyed and nervous. "I guess this is it!" she said.

"I guess it is." He put a hand on her shoulder. "You ready?"

Elle let out a big sigh. "Ready as I'll ever be," she said.

"Mommy, Mommy, Mommy!"

"Did they get there?"

"Did they get him, did they get him?"

"Guys!" I said. "Let me get my boots off!"

I'd barely made it into the house and my kids were all over me.

I said good-bye to my cousin who'd stayed with the kids that afternoon as I plopped my bag and briefcase on the floor. "Daddy texted just a few minutes ago and said they were on their way in—"

"What's her name?" Annah asked.

"Is he cute?" asked Caraline.

"It might be a *she*, you know," Annah chided her sister.

"Is *she* cute?"

"I don't know yet. They just got there after a really, really long day, so we'll just have to be patient a little longer, okay?"

"I'm hungry," William said as I picked him up.

"Me too," said Caraline.

Switching from work mode to mom mode that day wasn't easy. I'd been unable to get back to sleep after seeing Craig and Elle off to the airport. I was exhausted.

The witching hours were always hectic, but with no Elle there to moderate her younger sisters' bickering and no Craig to work his magic at the stove, I threw some frozen chicken tenders into the oven and called it a meal.

"Hopefully we'll get more news soon," I told them. "We'll just have to be patient."

I think I was more anxious than any of them. The suspense was killing me.

⌒∞⌒

Elle stared down a long, beige-tiled hallway, waiting and waiting as another woman stepped out from the doorway at the far end.

Craig pulled out his cell phone to capture the moment on video.

"Elle," the woman said, "this is Coach," and out came the most adorable yellow Lab Elle or Craig had ever seen. He was dressed in a bright-red vest. He was boxy and strong-looking, with the sweetest eyes and a face that instantly made them smile. His stride was almost regal.

Elle dropped down to her knees to greet him, as if all of her fear and anticipation and angst went right out the window. The handler let go of Coach's leash and that dog ran directly into Elle's arms, as if he knew this was his girl. As if he knew that's where he belonged.

"Hi, boy!" Elle squealed. "Hi, Coach. Hi!" She hugged him and scratched him behind the ears, and he pranced around like the happiest dog in the world.

"Coach? His name is *Coach*?" Craig said.

He was awestruck.

The fact that we weren't allowed to name the dog ourselves turned out to be a blessing, and in that moment, Craig was convinced that fate was smiling on us. That name meant so much to him. To all of us.

I had called Craig "Coach" back in high school when we'd first met. He was now "Coach" again to Annah's teammates on the volleyball team. Not to mention that Craig's stepfather, a man who had a thirty-year career as a high school girls' volleyball coach with the winningest record in New Hampshire history, was a man whom everyone, including his grandkids, affectionately called "Coach."

Being "coachable" and being a "good coach" to others was something we often talked about with the kids. We believed that to find a great coach in life was a gift.

That word had always resonated with our family.

"Can you believe it, Elle?" he said.

"No, I can't!" she said, cooing over that exuberant dog. "Hi, Coach! What a good boy you are. What a good boy you are!"

The woman who had served as Coach's trainer in Elle's absence asked Elle to pick up his leash and take him into the classroom, and the two of them followed her in with Elle firmly gripping Coach's leash. She expected him to go bolting into that room to try to go play with the other dogs. But he didn't.

"Now tell him to sit, and move your hand like this," the trainer said. Elle did, and Coach sat right away.

"Hey, that's pretty good!" Craig said, and Elle beamed with pride.

One by one, they were introduced to the others in the class—a veteran of the wars in Iraq and Afghanistan, a mom standing beside her daughter who was confined to a wheelchair, two teachers, and a teenage boy—with all of their dogs sitting attentively, just like Coach. Craig noticed that a number of the other dogs had been given girlie names, like Chanel, and he shook his head in amazement as he reached down to pet Coach behind the ears.

A few minutes later, the class instructor said, "Well, that's all for today."

Coach's trainer handed Craig a bag full of dog food. "We'll take some time to go over all of the various commands tomorrow. Just keep him on leash, and make sure he has food and water tonight. You also want to walk him before you go to bed, so he can do his business. Oh, and if you want him to lie down, just say *down* and point down, and he'll go down. He's such a good dog."

"Wait," Elle said. "We're taking him to the hotel with us?"

"You sure are, sweetie. The two of you have a lot of catching up to do. The other folks in the class have already had two days to bond with their dogs. You're his trainer now. He needs to get to know you."

"Oh," Elle said.

"We packed the portable food bowls and everything, just like you instructed," Craig said.

"Well, that's a good thing! You three have fun now, and we'll see you back here in the morning. Why don't you come a little early, let's say eight o'clock, so we can get a jump on things. You really do have a lot of ground to make up," she said.

Elle started to move toward the door, and Coach tried to lead her out.

"Uh-uh-uh. Pull him right back here now," the trainer said. "He is never to walk through a door ahead of you without you giving him a command first. So you tell him, 'Heel!' And you make sure he does it."

"Heel," Elle said in a quiet voice.

"Louder now. You're in charge, okay?"

"Heeel," Elle said. Coach still didn't respond.

"Forceful, like 'HEEL!' "

"I don't want him to think I'm mad at him," Elle said.

"He won't. He just needs to know you're in charge."

Elle took a breath and then said, *"HEEL!"* Coach instantly backed up, releasing the tension on the leash.

"All right, good! Now say, 'Let's go forward,' and go ahead and walk out."

Elle did, and Coach walked right beside her through the doorway.

Before they got outside, Craig stopped to take a photo of the two of them. Elle once again got right down on the ground and wrapped her arms around Coach's neck.

"You like him?" Craig said.

"I love him!" Elle responded. "He's awesome!"

We were halfway through cleanup before I heard my phone buzz on the kitchen counter. I rushed over to pick it up and the kids ran over, too, staring silent and wide-eyed. It was a text from Craig. *Finally.*

Suddenly, there it was: a picture of Elle with her arms wrapped around the neck of an adorable, floppy-eared yellow Lab.

I stared at that photo in disbelief. I couldn't believe this was really happening.

"Here he is," Craig texted. "And you'll never believe what his name is. His name is Coach!"

Coach? I thought. Of all the names in the world, the dog's name is Coach? I felt myself start to tear up.

I kept looking at that dog who was so impossible to imagine until that moment. I also kept gazing at my daughter, who looked so unbelievably happy and content and who had her arms so lovingly wrapped around that dog. I could hardly believe it. We'd been waiting so long without knowing what kind of dog might be joining our family. We didn't know its name. We didn't know if it would be male or female—

"Mom!" Annah shouted, breaking my stare. I looked up and saw all three kids ready to burst.

"You're never going to believe this," I said.

"What? What?!"

"The dog's name is *Coach*."

"What?!" Annah said, bouncing up and down like a kid on a pogo stick.

"Coach? Like *Grandpa* Coach?" asked Caraline.

"Yeah. Like Grandpa Coach," I said. "Can you believe it?"

"Is there a picture? Can we see? Can we see?" Annah said.

"There is," I said, pressing the screen to my chest and making them wait just a few seconds longer. "You ready?"

"Yes!!!"

I finally turned the phone around and my children lit up like it was Christmas morning.

"Oh my gosh!"

"He's so CUTE!"

"Hi, Coach! Hi, Coach-y!"

"Remember," I said as they jockeyed to get closer to the screen, "there's still a chance that he won't be coming home with them. So don't get too excited yet, okay?"

"Mom, look at that picture," Annah said. "He's so *cute*! That dog is *so* coming home. Even Elle's excited about it! Look!"

Annah was right. I don't think I'd seen Elle hug a dog since the first time she was bitten as a toddler. Yet there she was. Beaming.

"Well," I said. "We'll see. Let's get ready for bath time, okay?"

The bedtime routine that night took longer than usual. No one wanted to go to sleep. When all of the stories were read and all of the night-lights were turned on, I changed into my well-worn bathrobe, pulled my hair back into a ponytail, and lay down on the couch. It worried me that we hadn't heard anything else from Craig since dinner. I had no idea how Elle's blood sugar was doing with all of those changes in schedule and stress and activity. I vowed to stay up until I heard from him, but I couldn't stop myself from closing my eyes. The day had apparently caught up with me. I needed rest.

Just for five minutes, I thought.

⚭

"Did you send Mom the video?" Elle asked.

"I can't get a good signal. I'll have to do it in the morning. How's the homework coming?" Craig asked.

"Eh," she said.

Elle was sprawled out on her bed at the motor inn with her notebooks spread in front of her and that big yellow dog right beside her.

"I think he likes you, huh?" Craig said.

"I guess he does!" Elle said with a big grin.

"I was hoping he'd like me the best," Craig said.

"Well, too bad!" Elle laughed.

She looked tired, and Craig was absolutely beat.

"How're you feeling?" Craig asked her.

"Really, really tired," she said.

"Yeah, me too. Why don't I take Coach out to do his business and you brush your teeth and get ready for bed. It's been a really long day. You can finish your homework tomorrow," he told her.

"Okay. You be good, Coach," she said.

When Craig and Coach came back from their short walk outside, Elle tested her blood sugar. She was in range. "I had a snack before I brushed my teeth," she told Craig, and he thanked her for giving him the rundown.

Craig set his alarm for Elle's middle-of-the-night glucose check, turned the ringer off on his phone so his sleep wouldn't be interrupted, and then got up to turn off the light. Once again, Coach hopped right up onto the bed next to Elle, and she giggled. "Is this okay?" she asked.

"I don't see why not," Craig said as he kissed her good night. "Get some good sleep. I love you." Coach looked up at him with those big brown eyes of his, and Craig added, "I think we're going to love you, too, Coach," and he gave that dog another vigorous scratch behind the ears.

❧

The sound of the alarm on my phone jolted me awake.

I looked at the clock and it was 1:00 a.m. I could

not believe I'd dozed off for that long. Was my ringer off? I fully expected to see a long string of missed calls and texts from Craig as I turned off the alarm, but there weren't any. Not one. It had been hours. Where could they be?

I texted him as quickly as my thumbs could type: "Hey. Just checking in. Is everything okay?"

Craig promised me he'd check Elle's blood sugar before bed and text me the results. He promised to set his alarm for 1:00 a.m., just like I always did, to remind himself to test her again in the middle of the night, too.

It's not that I didn't trust my husband to take care of our daughter while they traveled. I did. I was just painfully aware of how hard it was to keep Elle safe on a good day, on a normal day, and this day had been anything but normal.

What if they fell asleep without testing?

I sent Craig another text: "Hope everything's okay. Just want to be sure. My alarm went off and I haven't heard from you, so please let me know."

I waited nervously for a response. I texted again. I poked my head in to check on Annah, Caraline, and William and found them all sleeping peacefully. I went back to the couch. I opened my laptop and tried to distract myself by responding to work e-mails. I texted once more. I waited another minute. Then I called. I got Craig's voice mail. I left a message: "Craig! Where are you? Why are you not responding?"

Pacing the floor at 1:45 a.m., I made up my mind not to wait past two. I told myself I would call the hotel's front desk if I had to. I'd get someone to knock on their door. My nerves tended to fray quickly whenever Elle was far from home. Trusting my instincts about her health and safety proved to be the right thing to do on far too many occasions. I had more than enough reason to disregard any fear of embarrassment or worry about inconveniencing anyone—especially my husband, who understood my constant worry all too well.

This disease was not going to kill our daughter.

⚭

Craig woke up with a start to the sound of a loud *thud* in the motel room. He was disoriented for a moment. Next thing he knew, Coach was pawing at his arm.

"What is it, boy? What?"

"Dad, what was that noise?" Elle said.

Craig turned on the light and looked around.

"I think Coach knocked your backpack off the table. Look," he said. "Didn't you leave it on the table?"

"Yeah," she said.

Coach stopped pawing at Craig and instead started nudging Elle's face on the pillow with his cold, wet nose.

"Is he trying to tell us something?" Craig asked.

Elle sat right up. "I don't know," she said. "Do you think I should check?"

"I think he wants you to," Craig said.

Craig pulled a lancet, test strip, and meter from Elle's yellow bag and checked her blood glucose—and sure enough, she was *low*.

"Oh my gosh," Elle said. "Dad, he knew. I think he knew!"

"Good boy, Coach. Good boy!" Craig said.

"Good boy!" Elle echoed, petting him thoroughly before grabbing some Skittles from her bag.

Ding.

"I'm so sorry," Craig texted at 1:50 a.m. "The alarm was set but I forgot about the time difference. We were asleep. You're never going to believe what just happened, though. Coach woke us up! He alerted!"

He what? I thought.

"He knocked Elle's backpack off the table," Craig texted. "The noise woke us up. I tested Elle's blood sugar and she was 68."

"You're kidding," I texted back.

To say I was skeptical that a dog was responsible for "alerting" them to her low blood sugar is an understatement. They couldn't have trained long enough that afternoon for him to alert already. How could a dog possibly know that Elle's blood sugar was low on their very first night together? And how on earth would he know to knock a backpack over to wake them up? It's a small hotel room, I thought. The dog probably knocked it over by mistake. It's a coincidence.

"I'm not kidding," Craig texted back. "We treated the low and Elle just gave Coach a reward for alerting. She's going back to bed now and I'll stay up to recheck. Everything's fine. I'll call you in the morning."

Everything's *fine*? Her blood glucose was 68, and they were there, and I was here. He knew how difficult it could be to get her back in range at times. How could he say "everything's fine"?

I took a deep breath.

I was very thankful that Elle was okay, and I allowed myself to feel thankful that the dog was there, too. Even if it was a coincidence, I was happy he'd woken them up before Craig's alarm went off. My baby was safe. That's all that mattered.

I made my way up to my bedroom and took one last look at that picture on my phone before my head hit the pillow. Seeing Elle's face made me smile. She was truly beaming, and it felt good to see her experience anything that could make her smile in that way. Coach was definitely hard to resist with his deep brown eyes and his adorably expressive face, too.

Still, I wasn't sure about this whole thing.

It wasn't until the next morning that the magic of what was happening in Kansas began to sink in for me. Craig managed to get a strong enough signal to text me the video of Elle meeting Coach, and I cried as I watched it. The catch in Craig's voice melted me, as he learned the dog's name and spoke it out loud: "Coach? His name is *Coach*?" And the sight of my daughter dropping to her knees and greeting that dog with such love and affection from the moment she saw him was heartwarming. I'd never seen her that way with an animal before. I must've watched the video twenty times in a row before I shared it with Annah, Caraline, and William, and they watched it another twenty times after that.

When I finally got Elle on the phone that morning during a break in their training, I could feel her excitement. "Mom, he's so *cute*!" She sighed.

Elle described how Coach snuggled up to her on the bed while she did her homework the night before. She told me again about the "amazing" moment when Coach knocked the backpack onto the floor as a way to alert them that her blood sugar was low. I, of course, asked if it could have been a coincidence, and Elle shot me down. "No, Mom, it's amazing. All the dogs do different things to alert—some circle, some nudge, some bark—and we'll be able to train him more if we want to train him to do something specific, but these dogs know. They just *know*. It's crazy!"

Craig described how he woke up to find Coach sprawled across the entire bed that morning, taking up all the pillows while Elle was scrunched way off to one side, almost falling off. She didn't seem to mind one bit, he said, and I could hear Elle laughing about it in the background as we spoke. I could hear her talking to that dog in a loving voice, the way I talked to her as a baby.

The more they shared, the more I could not wait to meet Coach and to see for myself what Elle was like when she was with him.

I had a hard time hanging up the phone. I suddenly felt very far away.

Elle quickly settled into her role as Coach's trainer during their first full day in Kansas. Craig was considered the "backup trainer," and they were told very clearly that Elle was the one in charge. It was *her* role to do everything that Coach needed in order to do his job well. It would be up to her to take care of his needs using structure and discipline to keep him happy and healthy.

Most of the training they dove into involved learning to master the basic commands: sit, stay, down. In some ways, it didn't seem all that different from what dogs might go through in a regular obedience class. And yet, there was a sense of importance to it. There was a weight to it. There was a mutual understanding that these dogs were going to help save the lives of every "trainer" in that room.

In the group setting, Elle and the other new trainers

worked on keeping their dogs focused, even while other dogs were brought in to distract them, or someone held up a treat, or when others in the class made lots of distracting noise.

"Down, Coach," she said as Craig held up a treat and tried to tempt him. "Stay." Craig did everything he could to get that dog to move, and Coach stayed right there. He could hardly believe it. He'd never owned a dog with that sort of discipline, and he never guessed that his daughter would enjoy taking on this responsibility.

"You're doing great, Elle," he told her, and she smiled and said "thanks," and got right back to work.

With the basics mastered, they turned their attention to some of Coach's more specialized commands. By saying "right" or "left," Coach would turn right or left. "Follow" meant he'd follow right behind her. "Hop up" and he'd bring his front legs up into her arms, or up on her lap if she were seated, or jump up into a car. Saying "easy" while he tugged on a toy would instantly get him to be more gentle. The "under" command would send Coach under a desk or a table and out of the way.

One command that really impressed Craig was "leave it." They could give Coach a ball, or even put a treat on the floor, and when Elle said "leave it," he'd leave it alone. Anyone who's ever loved a Lab knows that if it smells good and can fit in their mouths, it's in there. They're notorious for eating *anything*. Craig was like a kid watching that dog ignore a big treat sitting right there in front of him.

Coach could "tug" on command. If Elle told him to "bring it," he would bring whatever she wanted him to bring, whether it was a newspaper, or his leash for a walk, or her blood glucose meter.

He could even "shake" or "no shake" on command. After lying down for a while, dogs tend to shake when they stand up. It's not exactly appealing to customers in a restaurant when they stand up and shake and send fur flying everywhere, the instructors said. So all Elle had to do was say, "No shake!" when Coach was getting up, and he'd refrain from shaking.

"You're kidding me," Craig said. Of course, that line of instruction got him thinking. "So, you really want us taking him into restaurants?"

"Oh yes," the instructor told them. "For Coach to be effective, Elle really needs to be with him twenty-four seven. Especially in the first six months. That's why this training is so important. These dogs are trained to acclimate to work, school, restaurants, airports, just about anyplace you need to go."

"At school?" Elle asked.

"Oh yeah, of course. You spend hours and hours a day there. That's super important. You were planning on bringing him to school, weren't you?" the instructor asked.

"I don't know," Elle said. "I guess I hadn't thought about it."

"I think we were imagining this was more just for at home and at night, that sort of thing," Craig said.

"Does she only have diabetes at night or at home?"

"Well, no," Craig said. The instructor just looked at him and shrugged her shoulders. "Well, what about that?" Craig asked. "We seem to have all of these commands down now. Are there specific things we need to do for the diabetes?"

"Not really, no. You take care of Coach, and Coach will take care of Elle. That's pretty much it," she said.

"Well, how do we know if he's alerting?"

"You knew last night, right?"

"Yes," Elle said.

"Well, that's it. He'll let you know. You can work on training a specific response if you want. Some people like to train them to react one way for a low, another for a high. But the more you pay attention to him, the quicker you'll recognize it."

"And there's nothing else we have to do to train him to alert?" Craig asked.

"Nope," she said. "We trained him to do his job. Now we're training you to do yours."

Craig looked around as they all stood in a circle— at the war hero who'd fought in Afghanistan and now suffered from PTSD, at the little girl in a wheelchair who suffered life-threatening seizures, at a dozen other families who'd all come seeking help and relief just as he and Elle had. He marveled at how perfectly matched each one of the dogs seemed to be with his or her new family. All of them had somehow found their way to that church basement in the middle of Kansas. And every one of them seemed to be smiling, just like Elle.

Everyone else had been through two days of bonding and training with their dogs, yet Elle and Coach were keeping up at every turn. The instructors told them it was as if they'd known each other and trained together for weeks. They'd never seen anything like it.

The rest of that day was dedicated to grooming, which Elle would be personally responsible for on a weekly basis. Craig watched as Elle sat on the floor, brushing Coach from head to tail, brushing his teeth, using a special brush called a FURminator to pull out the undercoat that tends to shed the most, getting the gross brown gunk out of his ears and his weepy eyes, even trimming his nails, which made Elle really nervous. "I'm scared I'm going to hurt him, Dad," she said.

"You won't. Just don't go too deep. You're doing great," he said.

She *was* doing great. Craig loved seeing Elle embrace this responsibility. He watched as she listened to the instruction and took notes so she wouldn't forget. He helped her when she asked for help, but otherwise stood back and watched just how well she handled the entire experience. His little girl was growing up. Clearly, dealing with diabetes for the last five years had made her more responsible and responsive than the average twelve-year-old, because everything she did that day seemed mature beyond her years.

That night, Craig and Elle decided to go out to eat.

"You ready for this?" Craig asked.

"Yup!" Elle said, holding Coach's leash firmly as her father opened the door to a local diner.

"Sit wherever you like," a waitress called to them, and in they walked. With a dog. Into a *restaurant*.

Elle instantly felt everyone look at her and Coach, so she walked quickly to a table off in the far corner. "Down!" she whispered firmly, and Coach plopped himself on the floor with a sigh, curling himself up into a little ball.

"Well, hello there," the waitress said. "Where are you two from?"

It was clear that everyone else in the place was a local, and likely a regular. Elle and Craig would have stood out even without a big dog in a red vest.

"We're visiting from New Hampshire," Craig said.

"And I see you've got a new friend," she added.

"Yeah, this is Coach," Elle said to her.

"Hi, Coach!" the waitress said. "Aw, he's a cutie. He's from CARES?"

"He is!" Craig said.

"I love the work those people do," she said.

"So do we," said Elle.

"So what can I get you?"

Craig decided to eat like a local and ordered himself a very non–New England meal of chicken-fried steak with gravy, a side of breaded tomatoes, and Jell-O for dessert; then he settled in for some Daddy-daughter dinner conversation. Elle kept looking down at Coach, and they were both prepared to have to hold him back every time somebody new walked in or the waitress walked by with someone's delicious-smelling order, but he didn't move an inch, and he didn't make a sound.

The first outing was so successful they decided to hit up a local coffee shop for breakfast the next morning.

As they waited for their food, a customer approached them.

"It's amazing what these animals can do, isn't it?" the man said.

Like the waitress the night before, he was aware of CARES' work, and they talked for a while about the different dogs and the various services they provide. It seemed as if everyone in that town knew about the work CARES did.

"I wonder what it will be like to take him out to a restaurant back home," Elle asked after the man left.

"I don't know," Craig said. "I don't think I've ever seen a dog in a restaurant. Have you?"

"No!" Elle said. "I've seen someone with a seeing-eye dog downtown, but never a dog like this. Oh my gosh. Are people going to think I'm blind?"

"Ha! Possibly."

"Or what if they just think I'm some dog-crazy girl trying to sneak my pet in?" Elle said.

Elle was halfway through breakfast when all of a sudden Coach stood up under the table and put his head on her lap.

"Coach, down," she said.

He didn't respond to her command. He started pawing at her knee.

"Dad, I think he's alerting."

"Do you want to check and see?"

"Yeah."

Elle pulled out her yellow bag. Moments later, she had her result.

"Two-ten," she said.

"That's unbelievable. It's *unbelievable*!" Craig said. "Reward him!"

"Good boy, Coach. Good boy!" Elle said, petting him on the head and reaching into her coat pocket for a treat, which Coach instantly inhaled.

Elle corrected for the high blood sugar, and two minutes later Coach lay back down.

"Did you feel high before he alerted?" Craig asked.

"No, not at all," Elle said. "He definitely knew before I did."

"It's unreal. Wow!"

"Right?"

Elle told everyone in the group about her experience that morning, and they were all happy but didn't seem nearly as surprised as she was when it happened.

The agenda that Thursday called for a trip to the local correctional facility where the dogs had gone through their early training. The plan was to spend a couple of hours meeting with the inmates who'd trained them, and Elle was excited about it. She'd never been to a prison before, and she was hoping to meet the man who helped Coach become such a well-trained dog.

Once they were inside, it felt less like a correctional facility and more like some sort of reunion in a school function room. It was the first time the inmates had seen the dogs in months, and they all seemed thrilled to get to spend time with their former students. Coach's trainer, an inmate named Michael, was overjoyed when he saw that dog walk in with Elle. "Hi, Coach!" he said as Coach pranced around in his happy-dog dance.

Michael had trained a number of dogs before Coach came along, but he told Elle, "Your dog is the best. You've really got a special one." He said he kept a list of commands in his pocket that he used as a reference guide with Coach, and he pulled that piece of paper out and handed it Elle so she could refer back to it if she ever needed to. "This was my bible when I trained him," he said.

Elle looked it over, a printed grid with at least a
dozen more commands than she even realized Coach
knew at that point. Besides "sit" and "stay" and "down"
and "left" and "right" were commands such as "lights
on" and "lights off."

"Can he really turn lights on and off?" Elle asked.

"If you want him to," Michael said. "He'll jump
up and hit the switch. That's more for someone who's
physically disabled, of course, but if you need him to
do it, he will! We have even trained these dogs to strip
the sheets off the bed."

"Oh, I know!" Elle said excitedly. "One of the
moms in our group came out of the bathroom to find
that their dog had taken the sheets off the beds in their
motel room!"

She continued to read through the list: "Get keys,
get leash, get toy, get hat, get shoe, get pen, get *paper* . . .
get *socks*?" Elle said.

"Don't say it too loud now or he'll get up and try
to get all of those things at once!"

"What are 'open' and 'close'?" Craig asked as he
peered at the list over Elle's shoulder.

"Those are for doors."

"He can open and close doors?" Elle asked.

"Yup."

"Isn't that dangerous?" Craig asked.

"He'll only do it on command. If you were to

collapse or need help, I would say it's the opposite of dangerous."

"Wow," Craig said.

Elle thanked him for the list and tucked that piece of paper into her notebook full of handwritten notes about Coach.

In an aside, Michael told Craig that training dogs taught him that he could "do good for people."

Craig and Elle didn't know what Michael had done that landed him in prison. All they knew is what he had done for them.

"You be a good boy, all right, Coach? You be a good boy," Michael said as he petted him good-bye.

"I don't know what to say," Elle said. "Thank you. Really. Thank you so much. Coach is amazing. You did an incredible job with him. I really think he's going to help me in a big, big way."

Later on in the car, Elle started to cry.

"You okay?" Craig asked.

"Yeah. I just...I didn't realize this was such a big deal, you know?" Elle said.

"That was pretty special," Craig said.

"It's like we're a *part* of something really special. I just didn't expect it. I don't know what I expected, but..."

Coach poked his head up from the backseat and licked her wet cheek. Elle laughed.

"Good boy, Coach. Good boy."

⟨∞⟩

Back home, I waited anxiously for each new update. So did a growing group of friends and family who were suddenly very interested in hearing all about this medic-alert dog that I'd mentioned on Facebook. Something about Elle's journey struck a chord with people from every corner of our lives. When I mentioned the back-pack alert in one of my first posts after their arrival in Kansas, dozens and dozens of comments flooded in, and none of them were the sort of critical, doubt-filled comments I expected and had raised myself. They were full of "wows" and "amazings," and their words focused on just how wonderful this whole thing was and what a blessing this dog would be to our family.

I didn't completely embrace that feeling. In fact, with every new communication from Craig, I grew more nervous that a dog would just be one more thing to juggle in our hectic lives.

Then Craig hit me with news that I hadn't even considered.

"In order for Coach to do his job, he really needs to be with Elle twenty-four seven in the beginning," he said. "He needs to go to school with her."

"He what?!"

"You'd better call the school," Craig said.

Elle's principal and teachers knew she was going to pick up a medic-alert dog. We'd arranged for her to miss a week of classes and make up all of her home-work. Yet I hadn't given them any indication that this dog might be coming to school with her because it never even crossed my mind.

"Are you sure about this?" I asked Elle over the phone.

"I was hesitant about it at first," she said. "You know I hate the idea of letting diabetes define me, and I worried that by having him around all the time it would sort of be like putting a label on myself, which is one of the things that I definitely don't want to do! But then I realized that he's really, really cute and he's just a really good dog in general."

"Okay, but being cute isn't a good enough reason, Elle," I said. "This is a big deal."

"Well it's also because I'm his trainer," she said. "He's working for me, and I owe something to him. It wouldn't be right to leave him by himself at home all day. He wants to work."

I didn't really understand what she meant by that, but I called her school, and thankfully everyone reacted positively. Adjustments would be made. The school would adapt in whatever way was necessary, they said. I was thankful there wasn't resistance, but at the same time I worried about how it was going to work. If Elle didn't like having a little CGM monitor beeping in class, how in the world would she cope with walking the halls accompanied by a big yellow Lab? And what about the neighborhood car pool? Could we ask other people to transport a dog? Would their cars be big enough?

Then I reminded myself: There was also still a chance that Coach wouldn't be coming home with them at all. Coach and Elle still had to pass the public access test.

"What's that going to be like?" I asked her.

"They're taking us to a busy mall down in Salina," she said, "and I'll have to go through all sorts of exercises with Coach, making him sit and stay in a public place with lots of lights and noise and distractions of all shapes and sizes."

None of what she told me had anything to do with diabetes. It confused me. It sounded like we'd be getting a well-trained dog, which was great, but I wondered, *How will any of that help Elle or our family?*

"I just have to do my job so he'll do his. You'll understand once you meet him. I have to pass, Mom. We have to pass that test. We just *have* to," she said.

I told her that I was proud of her for how seriously she was taking this and how hard she was working. Of course, I had no idea how she and Coach were actually doing. I wasn't there. I was thousands of miles away, and that's exactly how I felt. I regretted not going. I felt sick that night worrying about whether Coach would make it home with Elle to join our family. The joy in her voice made me worry what would happen if they didn't pass. She'd be crushed.

I went to bed praying that she'd pass the test—even though I still wasn't ready for a dog.

⚬∞⚬

A video arrived on my phone in the middle of the next afternoon, with a note from Craig asking me to post it to Facebook after I watched it. So I watched it immediately. Elle looked radiant as she sat in a field of brown grass set against a bright blue sky. She scratched Coach behind his ears and in the most elated voice, she said, "I want to let everyone know that Coach and I passed our public access test with flying colors. He'll be coming home with us tomorrow!"

I called Craig.

"They passed?"

"They did great! You should have seen her, Stefany. She was so good. He was so good. Missing those first couple days didn't hold us back at all."

"How are you going to get him on the plane? He's not exactly small. Will they help you? What do you need to know?"

"They said he'll sit right under the seat in front of us. I'm not worried about it. He's not like other dogs," Craig said. "He's certainly not like any dog I've ever met."

I hoped he was right. Labs are big. They're bulky. They're amazing, yes, but they're rambunctious. I couldn't imagine taking a Lab on a plane when he couldn't be stowed in a travel crate. What if he had to go to the bathroom? It was beyond my comprehension.

I posted the video to Facebook, and once again we were flooded with congratulatory comments.

The next day Craig texted a photo from the airplane just before takeoff. There Coach was, curled up in a little ball at Elle's feet, tucked in snug like a piece of adorable red-vested carry-on luggage under the seat in front of her.

Okay. So maybe this dog was as well mannered as the CARES folks had insisted he would be. I breathed a little easier.

Then I realized what that photo really meant: *That dog is on his way to our house. He's going to be here in a matter of hours! They are all going to be home soon.*

CHAPTER 10

Little Miracles

"Coach gave me a reason to trust him. I know he can
tell when I need to check my blood sugar."

—Elle, age 13

I stood in the kitchen with my cell phone camera ready.
Annah, Caraline, and William pressed their hands and
faces against the kitchen window and jumped up and
down with excitement as Craig's car pulled into the
driveway. My heart raced as I hit the RECORD button to
capture the homecoming. I was just so grateful to have
Craig and Elle back home, safe and sound.

We watched as they got out of the car, then opened
the door to the backseat, and out came Coach.

"Awwww!" "What a good boy!" "Come here,
Coach!" the kids squealed, one on top of the other.

Elle led him up the stairs on his leash, and as soon

as she opened the door, her siblings fell to their knees and showered that dog with love. Clearly the little video clips I'd shown them from Elle's trip made them feel like Coach was a part of the family already.

"Sit, Coach. Sit!" Elle commanded. Even with all of the cooing and cuddling, he sat. "Down!" she said, and she pointed her finger toward the ground just in front of his face. Coach lay right down on the floor with our whole gang of children encircling him. They'd barely let him get two feet inside the kitchen.

Craig came through the door at that point and said, "What do you think, kids?" The kids barely even looked at him. They were too enthralled with Coach. Craig finally laughed and said, "Hey! What about *me*?"

I stopped recording and gave Craig a big long hug and kiss as the kids continued to gush over the dog.

Finally, as the kids began to calm down, Elle introduced me to Coach. I bent down and grabbed him behind the ears and looked into those beautiful brown eyes of his as I petted him.

"Hi, Coach," I said.

There was something calming about his face. His fur was so light it was almost white in the patches just in front of his shoulders and all under his neck and chest. He was sturdy, but soft and friendly, too. I'm pretty sure if I'd been given my pick of the litter, this is the dog I would've picked. In person, he was even cuter than he'd looked on my phone. He was perfect.

I was also struck by the power of the red vest he wore. This dog was on duty. He was working for my daughter. My daughter was in charge of him, commanding him like she was commanding her favorite role onstage.

"So the trip home went smoother than the trip out?" I asked them.

"Well..." Elle said, looking at Craig.

Craig gave an awkward smile.

"What?" I asked.

"Coach had a bit of an accident," Craig said.

"Where? On the plane?" I asked.

"No, at the airport. We should have taken him out for a walk when we changed planes. It was our fault. He basically dropped and did his business right in the middle of Terminal C at George Bush Airport in Houston."

"Oh, no," I said.

"It was mortifying," Elle said. "So, we really, really need to walk him before school, okay? I do *not* want that happening in the hallway. Can you imagine?"

"I'll walk him every morning," Craig volunteered. "Don't worry."

⚬◈⚬

Elle was pretty keyed up after the trip, and her blood sugar ran high for that whole first weekend. I could see

Coach circling her and nudging her hand with his nose, doing what Elle insisted was "alerting" her that she needed to test. Elle was accustomed to checking herself often during the day anyway, but I could see right away that with Coach in the house, she was checking without any annoying reminders from *me*. I was skeptical that he was really sensing anything, but anything that helped prompt her to check more often seemed like a good thing. Plus, the kids seemed to enjoy seeing him in action, and I had to admit that it was nice to have a dog in the house again—an eighteen-month-old, mellow yellow dog that didn't exhibit any of the terrible puppy instincts I expected to encounter.

When I went into Elle's bedroom for my usual 1:00 a.m. check on her first three nights home, I swear that dog just lay there on her bed and stared at me like I was a crazy lady. His eyes seemed to say, "What are you doing here? She's fine. Go back to bed!"

I liked Coach. He would sit and stay and was so gentle with all of the kids. I just continued to feel skeptical that he was actually able to detect changes in her blood sugar. On the third day, I called CARES to ask a few questions. I wanted to know if we should be doing anything differently or if it was normal for there to be an adjustment period after coming into a new home. I realized that by not being there for the training, I had missed out on a lot of information. I wanted to better understand.

They put me on the phone with one of Coach's trainers, and when I described the nighttime looks from Coach, the trainer asked if Elle had tested in range during those tiptoed checks.

"She did," I said.

"Then Coach is doing his job," the trainer said.

"Well, how am I supposed to know that? What if he's just not noticing? I mean, how do I know?" I asked.

That's when the trainer said something that sounded completely ridiculous to me: "Trust the dog."

Trust the dog? I thought. This is my daughter's life we're talking about. You want me to trust an animal with that? *Really?*

⁓∞⁓

Elle's first day back at school on Monday turned into a much bigger deal than we expected. The principal organized an assembly of all of the students so Elle could share Coach and explain what needed to be done to allow him to work during the school day. She was nervous going to school anyway, in part because she would have Coach with her, but also because she anticipated how some of the more "immature" boys in her eighth-grade class and others at the school might treat him, in addition to what they would say to her.

Elle was attending a small middle school at that point, with students from grades six to eight. Still, she wasn't prepared to walk into a room full of everyone all at once with Coach at her side. As soon as the kids saw the dog, they started swarming around trying to pet him.

"Okay, guys, okay, I get it," she had to tell them, "but you need to back off."

She was firm with them. I was impressed.

When everyone sat down, Elle stood in front of her whole school and explained how Coach worked for her. She also laid out some rules, starting with her insistence that no one pet him unless they asked her first. Her instructors at CARES had told her how important it was for Coach to stay focused, and attention from other people could be too much of a distraction for him to do his job. He needed to do his job in order to keep her safe so she wouldn't have a seizure or get really sick, she explained.

The kids were riveted, and Elle presented this information as if it was her favorite monologue in a performance. Speaking in front of a school group is very different from performing onstage, and yet somehow having Coach at her side seemed to put her at ease.

Elle went further, explaining to her peers that sometimes she would have to be really harsh with Coach. If he did something wrong, it was her job as his trainer to force him to do it right. To be strict with him. "So don't think that I'm being mean or anything," she implored. "It's just what I have to do."

She didn't want them to see her scolding and think, *What is she doing to that poor cute innocent animal?*

The transition from class to class went smoothly after that, other than a few surprised looks from teachers who would need to grow accustomed to having a four-legged student in their classrooms. The students followed her instructions and didn't try to pet Coach in the hallways. Coach lay down under her desk in each room and stayed calm pretty much that entire first day. Elle's blood sugar stayed in range, and he didn't alert that first day either. That was a good thing. All in all, she seemed happy about how their first day went. And if she was happy, so was I.

⟞⟝

I was startled by a wet feeling on my cheek. I looked at the clock on the nightstand. It was just after 4:00 a.m.

It was Coach's fourth night in our home, and his intrusion in my bedroom surprised me. Four o'clock is a tough hour for me. It's right in the middle of the only REM sleep I get after going to bed so late. I was so sound asleep that Coach's first attempt wasn't really enough to wake me. I dozed off again. Then two big paws pounced down on the edge of the bed, and that cold wet nose would not relent.

"What's up, Coach?" I asked in my groggy voice, half expecting him to answer. He just stared at me, eye-to-eye with his chin on my pillow.

I couldn't imagine anything was wrong with Elle. She'd tested in range all day. She'd had her bedtime snack and she'd tested within range just a couple of hours earlier. But up the stairs I trudged. I fumbled for her test kit on the bedside table, pulled Elle's hand out ever so gently from under the covers, and stuck one of her fingers with the lancet. The popping sound of that spring-loaded pricking device always seemed loud in the wee hours of the morning. It still surprised me that it didn't wake her up.

When the meter displayed a result, I rubbed my eyes to make sure I was reading it correctly. Elle's blood sugar had dropped into the 60s.

I rewarded Coach right away. "Good boy, Coach. Good boy!"

Did that really just happen?

I felt dazed as I walked to the kitchen to grab Elle some juice and a yogurt smoothie from the fridge. I put the straw in her mouth, tickled her cheek, and she drank. Coach remained agitated, circling around and pacing a bit while she slurped in a few swallows. I kept staring at him. It was shocking to me. This dog knew something about my daughter that I couldn't know. He came down a flight of stairs to my bedroom to wake me up and then stayed there and made sure I was awake— all to make sure that Elle was safe.

A few minutes later, Coach calmed down. I watched him plop on the floor next to my daughter's bed and heard him exhale. Almost like a sigh. I waited a few more minutes while he just lay there giving me that look again, like, "What are you still doing here?"

I retested Elle's blood sugar and sure enough, she was back in range. Coach knew it before I did.

I left her bedroom in awe. This was no coincidence. This wasn't some fluke. This wasn't some backpack on a chair in some cramped hotel room. That dog woke me up to tell me that my daughter was in danger. *And he was right.*

The next morning I threw myself into trying to understand Coach's capabilities better than I'd allowed myself to up until that point. I got back on the phone with the people at CARES and quizzed them about the commands and the training, asking questions about how best to make sure Coach had everything he needed to stay on task.

Even after making those calls, a full understanding of how Coach did what he did still eluded me, which was frustrating. I wanted answers. Even those who train medic-alert dogs don't seem to be able to offer a full scientific explanation for their abilities. It certainly comes down to their sense of smell. The difference between detecting scents in parts per trillion as opposed to parts per million is extraordinary. There were times when Elle's blood sugar was so high I could smell the sweetness on her breath. It's a faint scent, but almost as if she's been sucking on a lollipop. It made sense that a dog could pick up on that scent much faster, and it made sense that a dog could be trained to alert if a scent was particularly acute. Picking up on that sugary scent isn't a whole lot different than a drug-sniffing dog's picking up on the scent of heroin in people's luggage at the airport.

The baffling part to me was trying to figure out what the dog was actually smelling or sensing for the lows. Some theories say that the body produces more adrenaline when a person is experiencing low blood sugar, so maybe the dog is smelling the adrenaline. But isn't Elle producing increased adrenaline every time she's in dance class or up onstage? In the coming days and weeks, we'd see that Coach had the ability to sit idly in a corner without bothering Elle the whole time she danced or sang in a rehearsal. Then, every once in a while, he'd get up and go to her, circle around her, nudge her hand with his nose—and she'd test and see that she was either low or high and treat accordingly. What was he picking up on during those lows? And how could he be so accurate?

I still wondered at times whether it might just be coincidence. Elle came home from dance class one night and told me that Coach alerted, and she tested, and her blood sugar was 78. He'd been trained to alert if she dropped below 80 or spiked above 200. How could he notice such a small difference? I mean, *two points*?

It bothered me that I didn't know the answer. It bothered me that I wasn't able to find the answer. I need to see data. I wanted proof. Tangible, scientific proof.

∞

Coach continued to integrate into Elle's school and after-school life almost seamlessly. He maneuvered through the hallways and lay down under her desk in each classroom just as easily and peacefully as he'd flown from Kansas to Boston. He was welcomed with open arms at theater rehearsals, too. Sure, he had a couple of accidents that needed cleaning up, once in the lobby of the gymnasium as we walked in for one of Annah's volleyball games, which was embarrassing, but those accidents were entirely our fault for not making sure he went to the bathroom at designated times like he'd been trained to do. We were the ones who had to learn to follow the protocols. Coach was doing everything he was supposed to do. He would even go to the bathroom on command. He'd been trained to go as infrequently as twice a day if necessary, which I thought was quite impressive (and secretly envied). I had no idea any dog could be that good.

Elle's math teacher in particular, who had endured most of the annoying beeping of the continuous glucose monitor earlier that school year, told me, "It's just been amazing. I used to be so worried, wondering, 'Does she feel okay? Does she look off?' Now I trust that Coach is going to catch it, and I don't have to worry anymore."

I still wasn't quite as ready to trust Coach's abilities as some of her teachers were, but I also hadn't fully considered just how much Elle's teachers worried about her before Coach came into the picture. Somehow Coach's presence helped to break down barriers and gave everyone a chance to talk openly about Elle's condition.

At home, we all learned how to differentiate Coach's work time from his playtime by following suggestions from his trainers. We designated a work collar and a play collar, and Coach seemed to instantly learn the difference between the two. Of course, he always wore the red vest when Elle took him out in public.

On any given night, when the play collar was on, Caraline could be found playing dress-up with Coach. Annah loved to feed him and take him for walks because "Coach never tugs on the leash." William would sit next to him in the way backseat of our minivan or lie on the floor when he watched TV and pet Coach's silky ears like they were a suitable replacement for his blankie. In fact, all of the kids would pig-pile around him on the floor when they watched TV. I was stunned at just how easily he fit right in.

Craig followed through on his promise to take Coach for walks every morning, too. Before long, he'd found five different routes around Portsmouth's historic South End and Peirce Island, and those walks reminded

Craig of something he'd forgotten: His grandfather, a mid-coast Maine Yankee farmer, had instilled in him the importance of going out to "feel the weather" every morning while checking on the garden or bringing in wood for the fire. Coach gave Craig the excuse he'd been missing to get out there and accomplish that every day, without fail, and that made the start of each day a little better for him.

Elle was with Coach pretty much twenty-four seven for the first two weeks, and she impressed me with how much time and effort she dedicated to his care. It was as if she felt responsible for his well-being. I never had to tell her siblings to give Coach space. *She's* the one who told them to back off when they were climbing all over him. She was the one to stop Caraline when she tried to feed him food from the table, not me. When William tried to play tug-of-war with him, she intervened. "No, tug-of-war is a *reward*. Playtime is a reward. We have to wait until the right time to do that," she told him. She also let Annah feed him and help groom him, since she knew how happy that made her sister.

Elle took time after school to work with Coach on his commands, going through the list Michael had given her. I never had to ask her to do that. It was clear she liked to see him work, and Coach enjoyed doing work, and she wanted to make sure he was happy. On Sundays, she put him in the down position and sat on the floor to clean his ears and brush his teeth and trim the fur between the pads of his feet. You couldn't have *paid* me to do that at her age!

As a result, I didn't feel one-tenth of the burden I'd expected to feel when it came to handling a dog in our household. But it was way more than that. Slowly but surely in those first two weeks, I started to notice the moments when Coach would alert, and then Elle would check, before I'd even have a moment myself to remind her.

I knew that the more frequently Elle checked, the easier it would be to keep her blood sugar in range and the fewer long-term effects she would develop from diabetes. So that was a very good thing. I just wondered how long it would continue. After all, kids tend to get bored of things over time. Even things as exciting as a new dog.

When will the novelty wear off? I wondered.

The first time Elle left home without Coach was at the end of those two weeks to go to the mall with some friends.

"Why not take him?" I asked.

"I should do some things without him," Elle said. "After all, we won't be together twenty-four seven forever. And he does kind of slow things down sometimes, you know?"

She and Coach were supposed to stay together. That's what the trainers had told us. I understood her reasoning. I also wondered if maybe she was a little embarrassed sometimes to always have to stop and answer questions about her dog. Malls are crowded. She was sure to get stopped often.

It didn't seem appropriate to force her to take him. I wanted Elle to be in charge of Coach, and she had done a great job of it so far. So I let her go without the dog.

Coach was uneasy the moment she walked out the door. He watched her disappear with his nose pressed up against the glass of the kitchen window, just as our younger kids had done when they'd watched him arrive. Once she was out of sight, he wandered around the house and started picking up toys and things that he found on the floor. He kept bringing them to me and dropping them at my feet.

"Coach, what are you doing?" I asked, and he looked up at me with those eyes. "I don't have time to play right now."

He wandered off, found something else, brought it back, and dropped it at my feet again. He wasn't circling or nudging the way a dog who wants to play tends to do, and I knew because Elle had told us all firmly—play was only to be used as a reward. I looked at him again and it suddenly occurred to me that he wasn't asking to play. He wanted to work. He was used to working and he needed a job to do. I put a laundry basket on the ground and walked Coach over to one of the kids' stray socks on the floor by the couch. I pointed to it and said "bring socks," and he picked it up. Then I walked him over to the laundry basket and said "drop it," and he dropped it right into the basket. I did it again with another stray sock, and that was it. Coach was off and running. He started scouring the entire house from top to bottom, up and down the stairs, in and out of bedrooms and bathrooms, collecting stray socks (and a few of Caraline's stuffed animals) and throwing them in the laundry basket for me.

I laughed and laughed as he went about his chore. "Good dog!" I'd yell every time he hit the mark. I told Elle about it when she came home and I'm sure she thought I was crazy.

What *I* thought was Coach and I were going to get along beautifully.

We were just three weeks in when a noise woke me up in the middle of the night. I heard footsteps: the distinct *click-click-click* of a dog's paws on the wooden staircase and the shuffle of kid feet, too.

"Elle?" I called. "Is everything okay?"

"Yes, Mom," Elle replied. "Coach woke me up and I was 60. I had some Skittles and a little yogurt and I'm going back to sleep."

I nearly fell out of bed.

"Oh," I said, trying to sound nonchalant. "Okay, hon."

I wanted to scream, *"Oh my God!"*

Elle had never self-treated a low in the middle of the night. Ever.

Does she have any idea what a huge thing this is?

My mind started spinning over the possibilities that Coach had suddenly opened up for my daughter. Being responsible for a dependent child with a chronic illness, you rarely allow yourself to spend much time thinking about what will happen someday when you're not in the mix. It's too difficult to imagine, too worrisome to think that she's ever going to have to do this by herself. It makes sleepovers and summer camps and all of those experiences that kids are supposed to experience both traumatizing and painful.

A wave of revelation washed over me.

Coach wasn't just keeping Elle safe to give us some relief. He was empowering her with the independence she'd need in order to become a healthy adult.

I knew Elle wasn't going to be living at home forever. *Does this mean I won't have to worry every night she's away?* She'd be going to high school in the fall and then—God forbid—off to college in a few years. In that one instant, Coach made all of that seem less terrifying. Actually, he made all of that seem *possible*. I had not let myself think about how any of that was going to work since the earliest days of Elle's diagnosis.

I couldn't picture Elle at college, because I couldn't picture her getting through the night without my 1:00 a.m. testing. I simply blocked it out of my mind. I filed it away as something to be dealt with at a later date. Suddenly that filing cabinet in my mind was flung wide open.

Plus, it was 2:20 a.m. when this happened. I'd tested her at 1:00. She was in range then. What had happened between then and now? Had this happened before and we didn't know it? Of course it had. She'd had her seizure early in the morning. Was she on her way toward another seizure that night? Did Coach just save her from that?

I never fell back to sleep that night. I lay in bed thinking about what happened, waiting until morning to tell Craig about it. That was when it truly hit me: *This dog is going to do much more to care for us than we can ever do to care for him.*

CHAPTER 11

Coach's Spotlight

"My teachers are definitely more excited to see Coach than they are to see *me*. One even brought in a blanket for him today so he doesn't have to lie on the hard cold tile floor. Coach seems to like his new blanket, but I think he would rather get his paws on the tennis balls that are attached to the bottom of our chairs in that classroom."

—Elle, age 13

My Facebook post about Coach's feat that night brought an onslaught of love and curiosity:

Coach just caught a dangerous low and woke Elle up. I only woke up when I heard them together. Elle was rewarding Coach with a treat and she was treating her low with some sugar and it all happened without me. #thecavalryhasarrived

Friends and family wanted to know more. They encouraged us to provide regular updates on Coach and Elle. There was such an outpouring of love for this dog and what he was doing that it started to become clear to me just how much support surrounded Elle. So many people had been quietly pulling for her all along. Somehow Coach's presence seemed to inspire an outpouring of affection. People all over wanted to hear about every miraculous alert he made, so I started writing posts regularly.

A week later, I shared news of another alert:

Coach woke me up at 5:25 a.m. because Elle's blood sugar was low—55! So...Elle gets to start her day with apple cider and I start mine with gratitude.

In late April, I posted:

Coach is amazing! Last night Elle's insulin pump failed and he alerted two times in three hours because her blood sugars were high. After we fixed the pump, he woke her up this morning at 4:00 a.m. because she was low. I only woke up when I heard them returning from the kitchen together so Elle could treat the low with some sugar. This low was unexpected after she was high so much last night and I didn't even have to get out of bed. He has made our lives so much better.

Coach very quickly became a celebrity to our friends, but he also became a celebrity elsewhere. Just a few days after they came home from Kansas, Elle and Coach participated in Diabetes Awareness Day activities at a local school, alongside my mom and New England Patriots All-Pro defensive tackle Vince Wilfork. My mom spoke about her personal connection to type 1 diabetes with Elle, and Vince spoke about losing his father to type 2 diabetes at just forty-eight years old. It was an incredibly moving event, and Coach was perfect in a gymnasium full of kids all cheering and applauding for that big star from the NFL. A crew from our only statewide TV station at the time, WMUR Channel 9, covered the event and was instantly taken by Elle and Coach. The camera crew said they'd never heard of a "diabetes dog" before, and they asked if they could film a segment about the two of them for a show called *New Hampshire Chronicle*. I caught Elle's wide-eyed look of delight and instantly knew she was game. So we said, "Sure!"

When the *Chronicle* story aired in mid-May,

it raised Coach's local celebrity status. We'd walk through town to grab dinner, and perfect strangers would stop us on the street. "Oh! We saw you on TV! Is this Coach? Can I pet him? Or am I not supposed to?" they'd ask. Coach seemed to touch a lot of hearts.

The *Chronicle* cameras followed Elle to dance class, where they happened to film Coach alerting a low blood sugar. He got up from his quiet spot in the corner and came right across the dance floor to circle her and let her know that she needed to test. They caught Coach coming to alert me in the kitchen at home, too, while Elle was upstairs. He would always come find either Craig or me if Elle wasn't responding to his alerts. In fact, I was able to discuss a dramatic example of that happening in my interview for the story. A few days before the cameras came to our house, Coach came and circled me and nudged me, and I asked Elle if he'd alerted her, too. "Yes," she'd told me, "but I just tested a few minutes ago. I'm fine." A few minutes later, Coach went and found Craig and alerted him, too. Finally we both said to Elle, "Maybe you ought to test again, just to be sure."

Sure enough, with only fifteen minutes between tests, Elle's blood sugar had dropped a hundred points! She was down to a reading of 50. She didn't feel it. Elle never woke up on her own when she had a low blood sugar. She often did not feel rapid changes in her blood sugar at all. But Coach? Coach knew. And because he knew, we were able to get some sugar into her before she felt sick, or worse, and she recovered much, much quicker.

The TV piece included an interview with the principal of Elle's school, who noted how wonderful it was to have Coach at the school. He didn't bark in class, she said. He mostly lay there looking "a little bored," she added. She also explained how Coach once alerted a teacher that Elle needed to test after Elle had stepped out of the room and gone downstairs. I hadn't heard about that incident until I saw the piece on TV. The news was surprising to me, and I questioned Elle about why she would have left Coach in the classroom without her. She insisted it was only for a few minutes to run to the bathroom, and she'd stopped in the hall to talk to a friend. It was difficult for me to believe that Coach could alert when Elle was floors away; still, I was grateful that's what the teacher and principal had experienced. It was another reminder of the relief he was providing for the people responsible for Elle's care. Coach almost appeared to have superpowers in the television version of his story.

After the *Chronicle* piece aired, WMUR posted it on their website, and viewers from all over had a chance to watch and learn more about our experiences with Coach. One day, my mother was walking through the Capitol building in Washington when a visitor stopped her in her tracks. "Excuse me, but aren't you the senator whose granddaughter has that superdog?" We all had a good laugh over that one. Coach was famous, and my mom had become "Elle's grandmother."

Education, not notoriety, was the goal of allowing cameras into our lives. And we soon learned that Coach's forays onto television had a very real impact. A forty-two-year-old woman who lived alone in a rural New Hampshire town reached out to us. She had been struggling horribly with hypoglycemia unawareness for a long, long time. She had EMTs at her house at least once a month, and she wondered if a diabetes-alert dog might be able to help her. She had never heard of one before she saw Coach on TV. We put her in touch with CARES, she got on the wait list, and eventually, she brought home a dog. From what I've heard, she's doing well. In a very real way, in her situation, that dog could save her life.

The whole phenomenon was wild. Our friends and family got a kick out of it and were inspired by it, and Elle and I relished the chance to share our journey and especially to get feedback and support from so many different people. But I also worried that we might be sending the wrong message.

A medic-alert dog is not a cure for diabetes, just as a seeing-eye dog is not a cure for blindness. I didn't want anyone to believe that Coach was a cure for Elle's daily challenges. Coach couldn't make everything okay. It *wasn't* okay. In terms of Elle's condition, nothing had changed. Elle's blood sugar still seemed to suffer wild and dangerous swings for seemingly no reason at all, and while I was very thankful for Coach's assistance in helping us catch those highs and lows much quicker than we might have otherwise, all of our regular safety protocols were still required to keep Elle healthy, safe, and alive.

Elle began experiencing a new phenomenon as well, one for which I desperately sought answers: Her blood sugar started spiking on a fairly regular basis in the hour or two before she woke up, even after we'd done everything right. I wouldn't have known about it if it wasn't for Coach, and now that I did, my questioning of doctors and other parents of kids with type 1 led me to a frustrating conclusion. The cause of those spikes was most likely Elle's hormones. My just-turned-thirteen-year-old daughter's *hormones* could be causing spikes in her blood sugar. Yet another unseen variable to juggle. The most natural thing in the world, the inevitable changes that her body would go through for the foreseeable future, were becoming the source of a major problem.

Just before she flew out to Kansas to get Coach, Elle had gone in for another checkup with Dr. Ricker—and was crushed by news of her highest A1C reading ever.

She was 9.2. Elle was angry and upset and couldn't understand what she was doing wrong. Neither could I. I'd been nagging her about testing more than ever, and she'd been trying to stay on top of testing herself as it was. It was frustrating for both of us. It felt like all we were thinking about and talking about was her diabetes.

Now that Coach was in our home, we found ourselves talking about diabetes less frequently. The thing is, every time he would circle around her or put his paw up on her knee or sit and stare up at her with any kind of unusual attention, she would look at him and say, "What? What is it, boy?" And inevitably she would take out her test kit and check her blood sugar. I didn't even need to say anything. It wasn't that she was doing it to be safe, or because diabetes demanded it, or because she was afraid of having another seizure. She was doing it because she wanted to make sure Coach was rewarded for doing his job.

So much power came from her responsibility as Coach's trainer. From the first day they got home, her routine testing became about something other than diabetes. It was about her doing what she needed to do for Coach, as his trainer. That was such a powerful dynamic to watch. It was as if managing Coach's needs put her in control of her own health.

There was a heightened awareness in the dynamic

between them. It reminded me of what it was like to be a mother to a newborn baby. As you're getting to know your child, you find that you're painfully aware of when they last ate, so you're feeding them before they're even telling you they're hungry; you know when you last changed their diaper, so you know that in two hours you need to change them again, even if they don't feel wet. In the beginning you're so hyper-focused on the dynamic and the connection that you anticipate every need. That's how it seemed to be with Elle and Coach, with the side effect being that the more she cared for him, the more she was caring for herself.

In order for Elle to be effective as his trainer, she needed to help him maintain his focus, keep him in a routine, and make sure his needs were met. After all, he couldn't alert her if he was starving or needed to go to the bathroom. The net effect was that she was testing more frequently—not for me, nor for the diabetes, but for *him*.

Later that spring, I was struck by just how much things had changed. I shared the thought with my Facebook friends once more:

It occurred to me today that I have only received one call from Elle at school with a diabetes-related matter following Coach's arrival and it was on the one day when Coach was not with her at school because it was a rainy day and she was going on a field trip to a museum in Boston. Prior to Coach's enrollment in middle school, I would get calls from Elle every other day it seemed, reporting some problem... often a low blood sugar.

I am still discovering the remarkable impact Coach is having on our lives.

gratefuldiscovery

After five and a half years of dealing with type 1, I could say one thing with some certainty: We were doing the best we could. I was convinced of that. We'd worked with some of the best doctors in the field. We'd been through cutting-edge medical trials. We'd been fortunate enough to consult with some of the brightest minds working in the field today. And now we were working with a medic-alert dog who seemed to be having a real impact on Elle's life.

Still, was it enough? What if Elle's A1C levels were still not where they needed to be?

What else can we possibly do?

CHAPTER 12

Dog Fight

"This is amazing. I knew from the moment I got here that this place was meant for me. I want to be under those hot bright white lights. Sweating while I sing and dance and act on the scuffed black floor."

—Elle, age 12

It dawned on me in mid-May, about six weeks after Coach's arrival, that Elle would be heading to theater camp in July. She'd be gone for three weeks, to a place that she called her "home away from home." Her Oz. We'd made the reservations for the camp and paid the admission way back in October 2012, long before Coach was in the picture. Even after we got word that Coach was coming home, I had no idea what the dynamic would be like between them. I hadn't thought about the twenty-four seven nature of their relationship, and therefore we hadn't made any arrangements with the camp for Elle to bring Coach along. I'd assumed that Elle would simply go off to that faraway camp on her own, just as she had the previous two summers. I couldn't possibly have realized the strength of the bond and the dynamic between them until Elle and Coach were home. Coach didn't like it when they were separated for even a few hours. How would he deal with a three-week separation? How would Elle deal with it now that she was used to him? She was definitely more at ease when he was around.

I called one of Coach's trainers at CARES for advice, and the trainer's response was "No."

"No? What do you mean?"

"That would be *damaging*," the trainer said. "It would undo all the training you've already invested. Coach needs to go with her to the camp."

"Well, I'd be willing to work with him every day to keep him on track," I said. "I don't know if the camp will allow it."

"It's not good for the dog, or for your daughter," the trainer explained, "and they must allow it. The ADA law states that she should be able to take him wherever she goes. He is a licensed service animal!"

The word *damaging* kept rattling around in my brain. I couldn't let anything interfere with this dynamic between my daughter and Coach. It was going too well. I also thought about the added protection

Coach was providing to her, and I decided that it was more important than ever to send our canine insurance policy with Elle to that camp.

I decided to write a long, detailed e-mail to the camp director.

> I want you to know about a new development in Elle's life. After extensive research, followed by a painfully long two-year wait, Elle recently welcomed a service dog named Coach into her life and into our family. He's a diabetes-alert service dog who's trained to detect low and high blood sugars. Truthfully we were skeptical that this was possible, but our family was ready for a dog and figured we'd give this a try while we anxiously await advancements in medical technology. It's really hard to believe, but Coach is already earning his keep. On one of the first nights we were together he woke her up at 2:20 a.m. She tested and was experiencing a dangerously low blood sugar. Low blood sugars cause seizures. Nights are scariest for us when Elle is away at camp. Needless to say, we are relieved to have Coach providing reinforcement. Their relationship is just a few months old, and the next year is essential in making sure that they grow together. The trainers have recommended that they stay together as much as possible. Of course, we recognize that this may create added complexity at camp, and

we wanted to reach out to you to evaluate how we
might make this work.

The letter went on to explain how he goes to dance
classes and sits in the corner and doesn't move unless
he senses that's something is wrong. I explained how
Coach is an added backup for the safety protocols that
are already in place, and for which Elle had always
been compliant.

I included a link to the video footage of the story
that WMUR did about the impact Coach was having
on Elle's life, showcasing the interview with the head of
her school about the relief she felt with Coach around.
I explained that we didn't realize that Elle's separation
would be problematic until now. I apologized for not
giving them more notice, but I also explained how easy
it had been to integrate Coach into her school routine
and reassured them that I expected nothing different
for Coach's assimilation into camp. In essence, I tried
to explain it all.

I didn't really give the camp director the option
to say, "No, Coach can't come." After all, Coach is
a certified service animal under the Americans with
Disabilities Act. They couldn't refuse him entry or dis-
criminate against my daughter, and I was sure they
would understand that fact. This camp was very prestigious and had been in operation for decades. I imagined they'd dealt with other kids who had disabilities

and special needs in the past and I wouldn't have been surprised if at some point they'd worked with a child who had a seeing-eye dog. They were just that sort of forward-thinking and inclusive kind of place. *Weren't they?*

Much to my surprise, I didn't get a response. At all.

I reached out a few days later and re-sent the letter. I waited a few more days, then reached out again via e-mail and phone. Nothing. A whole month went by.

That's when I really started to worry. *What if they're not comfortable letting her bring the dog? What if that means she can't go to camp? She can't not go to camp because of Coach. That would certainly be devastating for her. The last thing we need is for Elle to resent Coach.*

I didn't want Elle to ever feel that the dog was a disadvantage or that he was holding her back, and I didn't want her to feel that anyone might think that we were now becoming difficult to deal with because Coach was around. Any of those outcomes would be terrible for her. I reached out again at the end of June, firmly asking for someone to please get back to me.

Finally I received a phone call from the camp director. She said they'd discussed Elle's dog, and then told me, "He can't come."

My stomach rolled into a knot.

Not only can he not come, the director said, but also the camp was no longer willing to have a counselor wake Elle up in the middle of the night, which was the protocol we had established in prior summers.

"What? We've already been accepted. We paid the tuition back in October. She's been there two summers in a row without any incident that prevented her from participating in the program," I said. "I don't understand."

The director said that Elle's needs were too disruptive to the routines of others and that they didn't realize that her routine would need to continue on a recurring basis.

"I'm sorry, but that's the decision we've made," she said.

"Well, that's not going to work," I told her. "This isn't acceptable. At all. Elle will be devastated. She considers this camp to be her home away from home."

At the end of the phone call, she said she would talk about it directly with the owner of the camp and that one of them would get back to me.

I was shaking when I got off the phone. I hadn't told Elle about any of this. I didn't want to worry her. I never expected this outcome. Not even close. I was willing to work with Coach and make the separation work if it came down to it, but for the camp director to basically say that they weren't willing to work with us on the simple task of making sure Elle woke up to test herself at night—that left me heartbroken. How on earth could I share that news with my daughter?

After that phone call, the camp director followed

up with an e-mail. "We've so enjoyed having Elle with us these past years that we gave this much discussion and thought. In the end, however, there's just no comfortable way to accommodate a dog."

I suddenly remembered something infuriating: That woman had her own dog at the camp the year before. Her personal dog! Her dog was there all the time, just running around and being a dog.

"Last year, the way we accommodated Elle was to wake her every morning at 1:30 a.m.," the e-mail continued. "We had no problem with this last summer because we wanted Elle to stay and we wanted to do everything we could to keep her healthy and safe. What I'm now reading in your e-mail is that this regimen may be needed again this year."

I wanted to scream, "It's a chronic disease! *It doesn't just go away!*"

She continued. "I have to tell you that I just assumed last summer was a passing phase in Elle's illness."

This is exactly the kind of shortsightedness and misunderstanding that Elle and I were trying to fight in our advocacy efforts. Preventing this kind of misunderstanding is precisely why Elle was so willing to share her experience publicly. Here it was, rearing its ugly head in my inbox.

Elle was one of their star campers. She'd won a Leadership Medal and was voted Most Outstanding Camper. How could they not want her back? I went to bed fuming, hoping that a discussion with the camp's owner would bring some resolution as soon as possible.

Finally that Sunday, less than a week before Elle's camp session was slated to begin, the owner of the camp called me back—and she was downright rude.

She suggested that if they allowed Coach to come, they'd have to allow animals to come from all over the place. "It would be a menagerie!" she said.

That, of course, was ridiculous. I explained, once again, that Coach was a certified service dog and that he had a right to accompany Elle under the ADA.

"The ADA doesn't apply to us because we're a private camp," she said. "Because we're an educational camp, we have an exemption from the State Board of Health."

That made no sense to me. Why would they have an exemption? Because they're an educational facility? Wouldn't that mean colleges could deny people with seeing-eye dogs? That was the opposite of what the ADA says.

It was insane to me, but I couldn't counter from a legal standpoint. I would need to research those laws to get answers. And I couldn't afford to get mad. I couldn't afford to tell her what I really thought at that moment. This wasn't about me. This was about Elle. So I bit my tongue, and I listened, and I racked my brain for any possible solution that might convince her to change her mind.

I reminded her that at least one dog had been there

the year before, who was just a pet. But she dismissed that notion because that dog didn't live with other kids in a dorm room.

"How are we supposed to handle the kids in her dorm room?" she said.

"How about you call them and see if any of them have allergies or fears of dogs. As soon as they meet Coach, it'll be a nonissue. This is a service animal. He doesn't bark. He works," I said.

"Where will he sleep?"

"He'll sleep in the bed with Elle."

"Where will he go to the bathroom?"

"You can designate an area. He goes to the bathroom on command. He eats twice a day, goes to the bathroom twice a day."

My easy answers seemed to only irritate her further, so she turned the discussion away from Coach entirely and instead focused her attention on the question of whether Elle should be attending camp at all. The owner of this theater camp said to me, "I can't believe as a mother that you would compromise the safety of your child by sending her away from home like this."

That's when I'd had enough.

"You have no idea what you're talking about," I said. "From the day she was diagnosed, the first thing I think about when I wake up in the morning and the last thing I think about when I go to bed at night is the safety of my daughter. To say anything otherwise is totally out of line. The only reason we even registered her for your camp is because when I called to inquire about putting her on the wait list years ago, after my daughter begged me for two years to let her come to your camp, the first question I asked was do you have twenty-four-hour nurse care? My child has type 1 diabetes. Are you equipped to handle a child with type 1 diabetes? I was told that you have three nurses on twenty-four seven and that you had accommodated other campers with type 1 diabetes before."

She interrupted me. She told me that there are summer camps available for kids with diabetes, run by hospitals that cater to their special needs.

"My kid *has* diabetes, but she sees herself as a theater kid. She doesn't want to go to diabetes camp. She said no to that years ago. She's *going* to go to theater camp. It's my job as her mother to empower her and try to prevent her from resenting the diagnosis that she has to live with every day any more than she already does and to ensure that she can safely participate in things that make her feel like herself. And isn't that what your organization is supposed to be about?"

There was silence on the other end of the phone. I realized this might well be my last chance to give Elle the summer she wanted, the summer she deserved, the summer she'd been so anxiously looking forward to for months and months. So I scrambled.

"Look, what if I was willing to set my alarm at

home and wake her up by calling her phone at one-thirty in the morning so she can test? What if she and I can manage that remotely, then would you let her come back without the dog?"

"If there was a way to do that without waking up her roommates, I suppose that might work," she said.

"She could wear headphones to bed, so I'd call and it would ring on the headphones," I said.

"Possibly," she responded.

It was crazy! My daughter was supposed to go to bed with headphones in her ears? I wasn't thinking straight. I was just trying to preserve some option for Elle. I could not let this door close on her.

That's where things stood when the phone call ended.

That night, I decided it was time to tell Elle what was going on. She'd already started packing. She'd been texting with her friends from camp and was excited to see them. It was time to put the ball in her hands and let her decide our next course of action.

I sat Elle down before bedtime and told her what had unfolded. I told her that they were not comfortable having Coach there, which was devastating enough, but when I suggested that they weren't willing to follow the previously established safety protocol, that's when Elle got really upset.

"Mom, do you know how many kids are on different medications there? There's a line out the door when I go to the infirmary. There are so many kids those nurses have to deal with every day! I walk right past that line, get my insulin from the fridge, and give myself my shots. I try to take care of myself as much as possible."

"Well, it's the waking you up at night that I guess they see as a problem," I said.

"It takes them two seconds. No one else wakes up. I don't understand," she said.

The pain in her face and the trembling in her voice was exactly what I'd hoped to avoid. She sat there rubbing Coach's head the whole time as he lay there, peacefully oblivious to all this chaos that was suddenly unfolding around him and, in a twisted way, because of him.

I told Elle that she could wear headphones to bed and that I could call her to make sure she woke up to test, and she looked at me as if the idea was exactly as ridiculous as I knew it sounded.

"No," she said. "No, Mom." Elle got a serious look on her face, and I could see the wheels turning over everything she'd just been told. "So what you're basically telling me is that they don't want Coach," Elle said, and she began to cry. "And they don't want *me...*"

I held her in my arms as she sobbed, and we cried together. Coach sat up and licked our hands. He kept trying to lick our faces, too. He snuggled his head into our shoulders until we couldn't help but laugh at his persistence. Laughing right through our tears.

"Good boy, Coach," Elle said. "You're such a good boy."

⌒∞⌒

The next day I shared the news with my family—and they all but unleashed the wrath of God. My mom was ready to make phone calls, my dad started researching the state law, and my sister in L.A. was ready to get on the phone to her publicist friend. They were ready to take this camp *down*.

"Hold on, hold on," I had to tell them. "I'm grateful for your concern, and I'm grateful because you feel protective and want to defend Elle, but time-out."

At that point I was angry, sure, but I was mostly just hurt that this camp didn't want my kid. I was hurt that my child was living with this chronic disease and had to put up with this *shit*! I needed to take time just to be sad, to take off my brave face while Elle wasn't watching.

In my heart, I didn't want to fight. I was raised by two people who are born fighters, who are advocates, who work for people who need and deserve reinforcement and support. I'm used to being in that position of fighting, too, but this was my kid. I didn't want to be the problem parent. Craig and I worked hard every day to not present her diabetes as a problem. We worked hard to minimize and redirect the worry and difficulties so that Elle could live her life as normally as possible. I wasn't sure I wanted to get involved in a legal battle that would center around Elle's diabetes.

After taking the bulk of that day to reflect on it, after listening to my parents, after looking into the issue of whether the camp was exempt from the ADA— which it very clearly was not—I finally wrote an e-mail back to the owner and director. I sent it on July 4:

> Thank you for taking the time to consider how Elle and Coach might integrate into the camp community this summer. Given our conversation on Sunday evening, I was forced to have a very painful conversation with Elle about this matter.
>
> I am struck by your unwillingness to work together so that we can find a way for Elle, with her service dog Coach by her side, to assist in fulfilling her medically necessary protocol to be a part of the camp family this year... I was hoping that we might resolve this situation in a constructive way that might work for everyone. Unfortunately, you've taken the position that Elle's participation at camp with and without her service dog is not welcomed by you or your staff. This position is unacceptable... We will be proceeding with legal action under the Americans with Disabilities Act. Please be advised that you will be hearing from our attorney very soon. Again, I am very surprised and sorry that we have come to this point, but your words and your actions have

made this about much more than a three-week summer camp experience.

A day later, seemingly *after* the owner and director
had forwarded my letter to their lawyer, they responded
with an e-mail of their own:

> I'm sorry it's taken so much time to respond to your
> e-mail, but we did want to give it our full attention.
> We've been proactive in contacting the State Board
> of Health to be sure we're in compliance with them.
> We've loved having Elle at our camp these past two
> summers, and I believe we've found a wonderful
> solution for Elle to join us again this summer.

It seemed they did not understand that they'd
already made my daughter feel completely unwanted.

"We've rearranged our rooming so that Elle can
live in the infirmary with the dog; that way she'll be
just down the hall from the nurses," the e-mail read.

So, I thought, *they want her to live by herself at
camp? Alone in an infirmary? Like some patient in a
ward locked in solitary confinement?*

> Elle will be solely responsible for the care of the dog.
> I do ask that we have all veterinary records and all
> the vaccinations and that Coach wear a service vest

so he's easily recognized as a service dog. We've
already begun writing up a protocol for Elle's care.

They went on to say that Coach would have to be
kept in a kennel the entire day and only be let out to
go to the bathroom. So even *then* they wanted to deny
Coach the ability to do his job. It was insanity. Dis-
crimination. Ignorance.

I still wanted to give Elle the chance to go to camp
if she wanted, so I showed her the letter. Elle felt more
disgusted and hurt than ever. "No," she said. "No,
Mom. That ship has sailed."

My last correspondence with the camp was to tell
them that Elle no longer felt comfortable coming back
to camp and that because they were finally trying to
accommodate Elle and Coach, we would not pursue
legal action. They refunded our money and we closed a
door on a chapter of Elle's life that had been one of her
most joyous.

Craig and I had done our best to cushion the blows,
to protect her. More than that, we'd worked to ensure
that she believed she could do anything she set her
mind to, despite her diabetes—that diabetes wouldn't
stand in her way. Now, in a matter of weeks, that camp
made the demarcation of Elle's BD and AD life crystal
clear to her in the worst way.

CHAPTER 13

Center Stage

"I'm happiest when I am singing and dancing. This girl's gotta do what she's gotta do. And Coach helps me do it. He's my buddy. He's a friend magnet. I take him everywhere. It's really, really awesome to have him."

—Elle, age 13

Sometimes when we're right in the middle of a fight, clinging to that thing we thought we wanted so badly or grasping for the one thing we think we want, we lose sight of the beauty of what is unfolding right in front of us. The fact is, sometimes our most difficult struggles in life lead us to the most amazing discoveries.

Once the tears were over, Elle emerged from her room determined to find a fulfilling theater endeavor to tackle that summer. Her resilience was inspiring to watch. It was too late for her to participate in any of the summer shows in our arts-loving community. Everything was already cast, and some shows were already up and running. On a whim, I looked at the website for Boston Children's Theatre (BCT)—and that's when I saw it. The Boston Children's Theatre summer program, a five-week intensive theater day camp held about a half-hour's drive south of us in Massachusetts, had a handful of open spots in her age group. They were continuing to hold open auditions into July, which was a first for them.

I offered to call right then and tell them our predicament, to see if they could squeeze Elle in, but Elle absolutely refused to let me do that. "Mom! No," she said. "I don't want you to call and say, 'All this happened. Can you make a spot for her?' No way. I'll earn my spot or not, like everyone else."

I admired her guts. I really did. "All right," I said, dialing my determination back. I looked into scheduling an audition. We spoke to the folks at BCT. We explained that Elle had a medic-alert dog. Their response was "Okay." They didn't hesitate at that news at all.

We decided Coach should go in with her from the very beginning, so in a sense, he was auditioning, too. They needed to see how easygoing he was when Elle took the stage. How patient he was. How calm he was no matter what happened in the room. They needed to experience it firsthand.

I couldn't bring Elle to her audition, so one of my cousins drove her down while I sat in a meeting, anxiously picking at hangnails while waiting for my phone to buzz.

Finally, it did. I excused myself and stepped into the hallway to take the call.

"Mom?" she said. "I got in! I got in!!"

"Wahoo!" I whispered loudly.

What we'd come to find out in the coming weeks was that Boston Children's Theatre didn't just *accept* my daughter. They didn't just *accept* Coach. They *embraced* them. The director actually wrote Coach into the musical they prepared that season: Coach played Bullwinkle the Dog in the opening scene of Act II. They placed a special sign on his crate backstage that read, "Coach's Dressing Room." When the group took an overnight field trip, they brought Elle and Coach along without any hesitation, fully accommodating their needs in every way.

Once Elle and Coach were on board, the directors used the experience to help inform and educate the entire cast. Elle talked about her diabetes. She told them all about Coach and the adventures they'd had so far. The trust Elle and Coach had in each other served as a model for how these theater kids needed to trust each other onstage.

Coach showed off his skills, too. I later learned that on the first day of auditions, he'd alerted Elle twice, helping her to catch two lows that might have gone overlooked until she felt miserable, or worse, had he not been present.

Elle came home night after night and told us about how wonderful the entire cast was to the two of them. I know that the love of that group was a trickle-down effect from the camp's directors. That's the way it works with great leaders and great teachers. Their students embrace the characteristics they embody—in this case their open minds, their compassion, and their inherent goodness.

On the night the musical opened, Craig and I sat in the audience feeling all of the same butterflies and excitement we had for any show Elle had ever performed in, coupled with a newfound nervousness about how Coach would perform onstage. I worried, of course: Would the applause throw him off? Would the bright lights cause him any distress? Then we opened the program and looked for our daughter's name, cherishing the moment like we always did—and found Coach's name listed right alongside the rest of the players in the cast list. We had two family members to be proud of that night: a dog who kept surprising us and a daughter who'd found a way to persevere and continue to do what she loves and to do it with people who embraced her for who she is. Fully. Truly.

Elle was happier than ever, and I do mean *ever*. I realized something had changed in me, too. That summer I felt a shift. I moved from a constant state of worry about my kid's chronic condition to a deeper, constant appreciation for my kid's abilities. Elle had become a powerful force for goodness in the world. She could *do* this.

Allowing Elle to grow and to embrace her life with diabetes was not easy. She'd managed to go through her BD life pretty much unscathed. The burden of her diagnosis and everything that came after it seemed unbearable. I think all parents want their children to live carefree lives for as long as possible, and it's a gigantic blow when that dream ends early. What I was learning to accept is that her life AD could be as beautiful as life before, and perhaps even more beautiful.

That night, yet another play in Elle's burgeoning career left me in tears from the moment the house lights went down. Only these weren't tears of fear or loss or devastation. These were tears of hope and gratitude and appreciation.

The lesson of that experience was huge.

When we truly surrender to what life has in store for us, it's amazing the beauty that unfolds.

Over the course of that stunning but always-too-short New England summer, Coach became more a part of our family than ever.

Bedtime had always been chaotic in our home. There were baths to take and pajamas to put on and bedtime stories to read and prayers to say and songs to sing—times *four*. The kids had always resisted bedtime, as kids tend to do.

Once Coach was around, though, he picked up on the routines and started making the bedtime rounds with us. William would go to bed first, and Coach would be right there, lying at his feet while we read him a story. Then it was Caraline's turn. Our resident little laugh factory would inevitably start speaking in a "Coach voice," trying to tell us what she thought Coach was thinking. Coach would then make his way into Annah's room, where he always got great big snuggles from the ultimate animal lover. Finally, he'd end the night in Elle's room, after she took him to do his business one last time and did her final blood glucose check before drifting off for the night. Along the way, our kids started to follow Coach's lead. They somehow didn't want to disappoint Coach by fighting their bedtimes. They knew that he liked to make the rounds, so suddenly the rounds became something they wanted to do for *him*. Craig and I were astounded at how easily the routines flowed with Coach in the mix. He had a calming effect on our entire household.

Coach also continued to show off the true depth of his skills as a medic-alert dog that summer—so much so that I couldn't fully believe some of the experiences at first. For instance, one afternoon when I was outside playing with Caraline and William, my dad walked into the house and took a seat on the couch. Coach came flying down the stairs and across the living room and jumped right into my dad's lap. Coach had never jumped on anyone. Ever.

"Coach," Dad said, "what are you doing?" Coach jumped off and started circling around and around, putting his paw on my dad's knee. My dad heard the shower running and realized Elle was upstairs. So he went up. He knocked.

"Elle, are you okay?" he yelled to her.

"Yeah! Why?"

"Coach is going crazy out here. I think he's alerting. Are you sure you feel okay?"

"Yeah, I feel fine. But hold on. I'll check."

My dad waited at the door, and a minute later Elle told him that she was more than a hundred points above range. She said she was almost done and would take more insulin as soon as she got out of the shower. My dad was stunned. I was blown away when he came out and told me what had happened. I'd already heard that story about Coach alerting the teacher at school, when Elle was supposedly out of the classroom and down a whole flight of stairs. Was I now supposed to believe that Coach sensed her blood sugar not only from downstairs, but also through a closed bathroom door? With the shower running?

It seemed impossible to me—until a few weeks later when Coach circled around me in the kitchen, clearly alerting. I knew Elle was in the shower upstairs. Two floors up. With the door closed. I went up and knocked. "Elle," I yelled. "Coach is alerting."

"Okay. I'll check," she yelled back. Sure enough, her blood sugar was over 300. She treated herself as I rewarded Coach. How could I continue to be skeptical when experience after experience proved Coach's abilities?

Elle grew so tall that summer. It was bittersweet to remember what she looked like as a little girl. I'd glance at the old school photos and family portraits on the walls in our home and shake my head at how quickly it had all gone.

She and Coach were about to enter high school, and Elle was definitely nervous about the transition. Portsmouth High is a big public school that draws students from a number of surrounding towns. There would be nearly a thousand kids in those halls, including hundreds and hundreds of perfect strangers.

Elle would turn fourteen that September, which put her on the younger end of the spectrum compared to many of her classmates. I could tell she was nervous about the social aspects of it just from how selective she was with the choices she made as we went about our back-to-school shopping. And it was on that shopping trip that she casually mentioned how hard it would be to blend in walking the halls with a big yellow dog in a red vest at her side.

Before I knew it, off she went. My first baby. A freshman. I remember being a high school freshman like it was yesterday. Craig and I both joked about how old it made us feel. How on earth did we have a daughter in high school?

Late that September, it came time for Elle to go in for a routine checkup at Joslin Diabetes Center. She had missed a scheduled checkup over the summer because of theater camp. So we were going on six months since her last appointment with her endocrinologist, and I was dreading it because the results of her last A1C tests were still weighing on us.

So much had gone so well since Coach came along, other than the theater camp fiasco—and even that turned out well for Elle in the end. Coach had been helping us catch highs and lows left and right. We were approaching yet another year without a seizure. So naturally we both started to grow anxious that an inevitable shoe would drop.

If Elle's A1C levels still are elevated, what are we going to do?

CHAPTER 14

Super Dog

"Having Coach is like a sigh of relief because now I know that this actually works, and it is going to be an amazing journey for both of us and for my whole family."

—Elle, age 13

So," Dr. Ricker asked, "why choose a dog over a continuous glucose monitor?"

Coach lay quietly on the floor, sleepily conspicuous in his bright-red vest, as Elle sat on the edge of the examination table.

"Well," Elle said, "I really don't have to choose. I may do both. But Coach is very cuddly, and I can't snuggle up with a continuous glucose monitor the way I can with Coach."

Dr. Ricker laughed. We'd been through a lot with this woman, and I'm not sure I'd ever heard her laugh.

Dr. Ricker had recently informed us that she would soon be retiring, which saddened us. The close-knit medical circle you depend on with a chronic illness really does become like an extended family. The thought of losing a member of the team was painful. We wouldn't have many more visits with her.

"What are some of the significant differences you've experienced now that you have Coach?" she asked Elle.

"I'm definitely more tuned in to when I need to be checking blood sugars," Elle said. The doctor seemed impressed.

Then Elle revealed something I didn't see coming. "And," she said, "you know, having Coach—it feels like the first time diabetes has given something back to my family instead of just taking things away."

It still shocked me how much Elle had internalized some of her feelings about this disease. For such an outgoing kid, she kept a lot inside. It was heartbreaking for me to hear her say out loud that she thought diabetes had taken so much away from her family; at the same time it felt gratifying to hear her acknowledge the impact Coach was having on our family.

The doctor went about her exam while we waited for the results of Elle's A1C test to come back. The 9.2 from her previous visit felt like a giant elephant in the room. Elle hadn't had a single reading in the desired

7 to 7.5 range since she hit her preteen years. We'd discussed it on the drive down that day, and we agreed that just getting her back down into the 8s would be a big victory.

Elle took my hand as Dr. Ricker pulled up the results on her computer.

"Wow," Dr. Ricker said. "Elle?"

"Yeah?"

"Your A1C is 7.2."

"It *is*?" Elle said.

"It is!" Dr. Ricker said. She was exuberant. "That's wonderful news!"

Elle's face lit up and she gave me a big high five. "Yes, Mom!" she shouted.

That A1C number wasn't just wonderful. It was the lowest A1C she'd ever had. Elle was still at the height of puberty, perhaps the most difficult time for controlling blood sugars. That number was a huge victory, and the doctor agreed wholeheartedly.

Elle jumped down to the floor.

"See, Coach! It's working. You're working!" she said. She rubbed his ears, and he groaned. Coach groaned or moaned at the funniest times, like he was just so exasperated by how slow we were to realize his many gifts. He looked at us like, "Yeah, yeah, I know it's working. What did you expect?"

Once again, I found myself in awe. Other than Coach's presence, nothing else had changed to lead Elle toward this result. If anything, I half expected her A1C to be worse because of her recent growth spurt.

Coach was the only possible explanation. This wasn't anecdotal evidence that he *seemed* to be having a positive effect on Elle's health. This was verifiable evidence that Elle was doing significantly better because of Coach's presence. The data spoke for itself.

I do not mean to suggest that a dog like Coach can work for everyone with type 1. Research on a broader population is required and our experience is not "proof." This result for Elle could just mean that Coach is having the effect of encouraging her to test more frequently, so she has more of an opportunity to treat highs and lows. Maybe that's all it is. Maybe there isn't anything particularly magical about Coach and his abilities. But it doesn't matter to me. To us. The result is the same. Whether Coach is right all the time or not, the result is she's testing more frequently and she's catching things when she needs to be, not when she's feeling miserable and is already too high or too low.

Still, in our own experience, more often than not, Coach is *right*. If he was wrong all the time, his effectiveness would surely fade because she wouldn't be incentivized to keep testing. Coach is *right*. Over and over again, under the most amazing circumstances, he's *right*.

⌘

As Elle's high school schedule kicked into high gear, she and I started spending less time together. There were mornings when she'd be up at 5:30, go off to school, and wouldn't come home from after-school activities until 5:30 at night. Then she'd often have play rehearsals or something until bedtime.

Throughout it all, Elle leaned on Coach. I leaned on Coach, too. Coach gave so much to both of us that it actually allowed Elle and me to get back to being mom and daughter again instead of the exhausted caregiver and the aggravated patient.

I suppose her wonderful A1C result just reinforced what I was already feeling.

I was feeling some relief.

Of course, I will always be a big believer in the potential for science and modern medicine to fundamentally change my daughter's life for the better and one day cure diabetes. I will always search for proof of the potential for new treatments and technologies. But for now, Elle's physical and emotional health was all the evidence I needed. From that point forward, I was finally able to do what the trainer had told me to do at the very beginning: "Trust the dog."

Elle and Coach and I formed a sort of three-legged stool now. Each leg depended on the other, and the trust we'd built in each other provided the strength we needed to stand tall.

It was amazing to me how quickly my faith in Coach freed up some room in my heart to focus on other areas of my own life. That fall I decided it was time for me to give back to the community that gave my family so much. I wanted to do what I could to help shape the future of the city my family called home. So following in my mom's footsteps, and with the full support of Craig and the kids, I threw my hat into the political ring for the first time. I decided to run for a seat on the Portsmouth city council.

I dove headfirst into the process, attacking it with the energy with which I attack everything. Craig and the kids and Coach often canvassed with me as I knocked on more than a thousand doors, shaking hands, handing out postcards, and putting up signs. Their presence helped me when it came time for voters to go to the polls. My family was everything to me. They were my motivation and inspiration. And it showed.

Coach and Elle happened to be in the van with Craig and me when my phone rang on election night. We were all together when I got the news.

I won.

We threw a victory celebration that night. So many loved ones were there. Friends, parents, all of our kids, good music, good food—and Coach sitting quietly in the corner, keeping his watchful eye on my oldest girl as she danced the night away.

As Christmas Eve came around, Coach decided to get in on the dancing himself. Caraline pulled up Pandora and put on some Motown as we all assembled a gingerbread house together in the kitchen. That's when Coach jumped his front paws right into Elle's arms. They danced together. Suddenly everyone wanted a turn dancing with Coach. Annah jumped in, then Caraline, then William, then Craig. I finally took his paws and danced with him, too—that beautiful dog who'd done so much for our family. Then Elle grabbed one paw as I held the other, and the three of us danced together. I swear that amazing yellow Lab was smiling just as broadly as we were.

That winter started early and seemed to stretch on forever, and it was particularly cold the first time it happened.

Elle was frantically behind schedule, gathering up her things and getting ready to run across town to a theater rehearsal. The wind was whipping, blowing white wisps of shimmering snowflakes from the rooftops in the late-afternoon glow of the setting sun. Craig was busy making dinner for the rest of the family when she and Coach went running past us.

"Bye, Mom! Bye, Dad!" she yelled as the wind whipped in.

"Bye. Shut the door! Quick!" I called after her.

Ten minutes later, I caught it.

I stopped what I was doing and looked out the window. I realized I'd let Elle go without saying a word. I didn't run through the safety checklist. I didn't make her sit down and test. I didn't ask her what she'd eaten. I didn't check her coat pockets to make sure she had Skittles. None of it.

I'd let her go without a word—and I wasn't panicked.

I knew that my daughter was going to be okay.

I would never stop worrying, of course. What mother ever does? But in that moment, for the very first time since it all began, I finally felt calm—because I knew that Elle had her Coach.

AFTERWORD

"If we work together, our leaders will see how important it is that we find a cure."

—Elle, age 12

On November 29, 2013, I wrote the following post on my Facebook page:

Six years ago today Elle was diagnosed with type 1 diabetes. To date, she has pricked her fingers to test her blood sugar nearly 22,000 times and taken more than 10,000 shots. She has endured 5 hospital stays and participated in 4 medical research trials. Not to mention the countless number of sleepless nights. By the numbers, diabetes has had an impressive impact. And all the little moments that this diagnosis endlessly steals from our lives really add up. So on this, the 2,190th day of life with diabetes, I am going to count on the doctors, researchers, inventors, advocates, and families who are fighting tirelessly for a day without diabetes!

As much as we've come to count on Coach in our day-to-day lives, it really is the researchers, inventors, doctors, and advocates whom we count on the most.

According to CARES, the working life of a medic-alert dog is only about ten years. Their sense of smell and their overall alertness diminishes pretty quickly after a decade.

Elle had the chance to meet with Dean Kamen after Coach came into our lives. He was interested to hear every detail of Coach's story and was so happy that we were finding some relief. But when Elle told him that Coach's effectiveness had an expiration date, she also gave him an ultimatum.

"I've had Coach over a year already," she said. "So that means you only have about eight years left to find a cure or some other solution to this, okay? I don't want to get another service dog. I want a cure."

Dean smiled at Elle's moxie, and then he reached out to shake my daughter's hand. "You've got it," he said. "I'll do everything I can."

I believe him. I believe that all the doctors and

scientists we've met along the way are working with everything they have to put an end to this disease, and I know that they are getting closer every day. I also know that there will be small improvements in the meantime. There's a new generation of continuous glucose monitors on the market now, and Elle is having much more success using this new device than she did with the early-generation model a few years ago. It's one more bit of support that will help her to monitor her blood sugar. And yet, that is still no cure. It's up to all of us to keep fighting for the funding scientists and researchers need in order to succeed. It is up to us to keep fighting for regulatory pathways to ensure that better treatments reach the marketplace.

My job as Elle's mother is to raise her to be an independent, self-sufficient, contributing member of society. Wrestling with the reality that my child might not be able to be as independent as she wants or needs to be was heartbreaking. Coach healed my heartbreak. I've lost count of how many times he's woken her up in the middle of the night now and how many times she's tested and treated herself because of him.

Every time Coach catches a low or a high for Elle, it amazes me. My gratitude for what he's doing for my daughter and for our family is immeasurable.

Coach may not be a cure, but he provides tremendous comfort, reassurance, and reinforcement while the journey toward a cure continues.

It's remarkable, isn't it? Sometimes having faith in something, even something we don't fully understand, makes us stronger than we were before. It is in faith that we find hope—the hope that we can rise up to tomorrow no matter what life brings.

ACKNOWLEDGMENTS

This book—and our story itself—would not have been possible without the support and inspiration of so many. I could not resist the opportunity and I hope you will indulge me while I celebrate those who mean the world to me.

Elle, Annah, Caraline, and William, who taught me how to love unconditionally and who inspire me every day.

Craig, who makes it all possible.

My parents, who set the bar incredibly high and taught me how to reach for the stars.

My sisters, Stacey and Molly, who keep me honest and made me ferociously protective.

Nikki Hill, for loving my children like her own. And for all of my cousins, who are there in the good times and the bad times.

Aunt Mary McKinnon, for planting the seed of confidence in me that I could write a book when I was just a little girl. And for my aunt Peggy Fennelly and our extended family, for teaching us the importance of the legacy we are part of and the responsibility we share to carry it forward.

My brother-in-law, Trent Welch, for sharing this

diabetes journey with us and for being our emergency hotline in those early days following Elle's diagnosis.

My oldest and dearest friends, Ambre, Amy, Jill, Sara, and Timmie, who love me for me.

My teammate through so many adventures and challenges, Stacey Pascarella Swineford, for being the family we choose.

Our first friends as a couple, Anna Kay Vorsteg and Vicki Boyd, for reminding us to be courageous through all of life's passages.

Coach and Ellen Garneau, for giving Craig to me.

George Bennett, for believing in me.

Mary Jo Brennan, for encouraging me every step of the way.

Joslin Diabetes Center, for taking care of Elle.

JDRF, for leading the tireless campaign for a cure and better treatment year after year.

My favorite high school English teacher, Liz Whaley, for teaching me how to write.

Dean Kamen, who gives us reason to hope.

Mark Dagostino, for his compassion, patience, and tireless dedication to telling our story with authenticity and integrity.

The team at Hachette, for helping us bring this story to life. I would especially like to thank Mauro DiPreta, for taking a chance on me; Michelle Aielli, for making sure people find out about this book; and Betsy Hulsebosch, for making sure people have a chance to buy this book.